JOHN MUIR
TRAIL
— DATA BOOK —

T0020888

Elizabeth Wenk

WILDERNESS PRESS . . . *on the trail since 1967*

John Muir Trail Data Book

First edition, 2014; second edition, 2022
Copyright © 2014, 2022 by Keen Communications

Project editor: Ritchey Halphen
Cover design: Scott McGrew
Cartography: Elizabeth Wenk
Text design: Andreas Schüller, with updates by Annie Long
Photos: © Elizabeth Wenk, except as noted

Library of Congress Cataloging-in-Publication Data is available at catalog.loc.gov.
ISBN 978-1-64359-093-6 (pbk.) | ISBN 978-1-64359-094-3 (ebook)

WILDERNESS PRESS
An imprint of AdventureKEEN
2204 First Ave. S., Ste. 102
Birmingham, AL 35233
800-678-7006, fax 877-374-9016

Manufactured in the United States of America
Distributed by Publishers Group West

Cover photo: Camping in the Sierra Nevada; © Patrick Poendl/Shutterstock

Visit wildernesspress.com for a complete listing of our books and for ordering information. Contact us at our website, at facebook.com/wildernesspress1967, or at twitter.com/wilderness1967 with questions or comments. To find out more about who we are and what we're doing, visit blog.wilderness press.com.

SAFETY NOTICE Although Wilderness Press and the author have made every attempt to ensure that the information in this book is accurate at press time, they are not responsible for any loss, damage, injury, or inconvenience that may occur while using this book. You are responsible for your own safety and health while in the wilderness. The fact that a trail is described in this book does not mean that it will be safe for you. Be aware that trail conditions can change from day to day. Always check local conditions, know your own limitations, and consult a map.

Contents

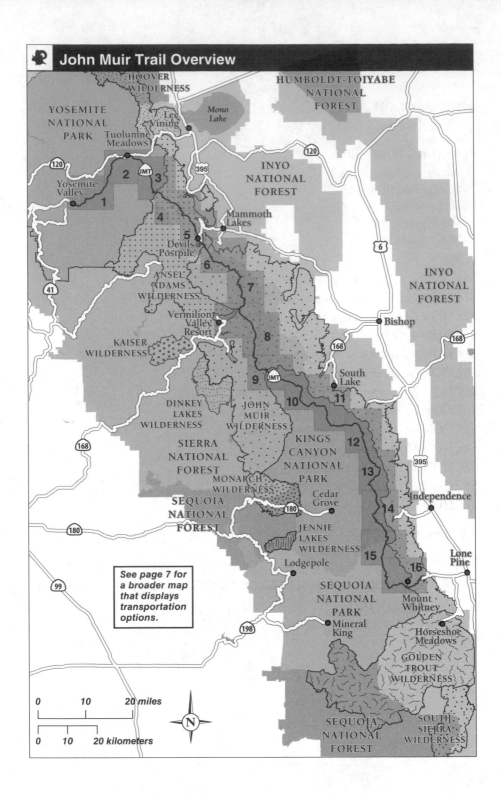

John Muir Trail Overview

HOOVER WILDERNESS

HUMBOLDT-TOIYABE NATIONAL FOREST

YOSEMITE NATIONAL PARK

Mono Lake

Lee Vining

Tuolumne Meadows

120

2

JMT

3

2

395

INYO NATIONAL FOREST

120

Yosemite Valley

1

4

Mammoth Lakes

5

Devils Postpile

6

41

ANSEL ADAMS WILDERNESS

7

6

INYO NATIONAL FOREST

Vermilion Valley Resort

8

Bishop

KAISER WILDERNESS

168

DINKEY LAKES WILDERNESS

9

JMT

South Lake

10

168

11

JOHN MUIR WILDERNESS

SIERRA NATIONAL FOREST

KINGS CANYON NATIONAL PARK

12

168

MONARCH WILDERNESS

13

395

SEQUOIA NATIONAL FOREST

Cedar Grove

14

Independence

180

180

JENNIE LAKES WILDERNESS

15

Lone Pine

99

Lodgepole

16

Mount Whitney

See page 7 for a broader map that displays transportation options.

SEQUOIA NATIONAL PARK

Horseshoe Meadows

198

Mineral King

GOLDEN TROUT WILDERNESS

0   10   20 miles

0   10   20 kilometers

N

SEQUOIA NATIONAL FOREST

SOUTH SIERRA WILDERNESS

Introduction

The John Muir Trail—or, more simply, the JMT—is one of the world's premier long-distance hiking trails. A little more than 220 miles in length, it traverses the spine of California's Sierra Nevada, passing through superb mountain scenery. This is a land of 13,000- and 14,000-foot peaks, of soaring granite cliffs, of lakes by the thousands, and of canyons 5,000 feet deep. The trail passes near roads only in Tuolumne Meadows and Devils Postpile, otherwise winding through remote mountain landscapes.

Part of the beauty of this long-distance walk is that the landscape continually changes as you travel from Happy Isles (in eastern Yosemite Valley) to Whitney Portal (west of the town of Lone Pine, in the Owens Valley). Each day you will find new wonders to captivate your attention: rounded domes in Tuolumne Meadows, volcanic features near Devils Postpile, magical hemlock forests near Silver Pass, dashing cascades along Bear Creek, the glacial landscape of Evolution Basin, the near-vertical peaks of the Palisades, carpets of alpine flowers around Pinchot Pass, spectacular lake basins such as the Rae Lakes, scattered foxtail pines on Bighorn Plateau, and of course the views from the summit of Mount Whitney, California's tallest peak.

The Sierra is an especially lovely area for a multiweek hike, for it is blessed with the mildest, sunniest climate of any major mountain range in the world. Though rain does fall in the summer, it seldom lasts more than an hour or two, and the sun is out and shining most hours of the day. Most likely, the greatest challenge you will face is the logistics of resupplying food because the southern 160 miles do not pass a road, and for the final 110 miles you do not even pass close to a food resupply "depot." You are, of course, not the only person to have heard of these attractions and will encounter people daily, but the trail really is a thin line through a vast land; with little effort you can always camp on your own if you leave the trail.

Using This Book

This book is a companion to *John Muir Trail: The Essential Guide to Hiking America's Most Famous Trail,* also published by Wilderness Press. As the title indicates, the *Data Book* focuses exclusively on the data sections of the larger book, including tables with junction locations and distances between junctions, topographic maps, elevation profiles, a table of campsite locations, and some basic information to help you plan your trip.

If you are seeking trail descriptions, information about natural history of the region, suggestions for possible side trips along the trail, or advice on how to hike in the Sierra, I recommend that you purchase the thicker volume. If, however, you anticipate it will be too heavy for the trail, carry a copy of this book instead.

This guide provides you with the data you need to design your own trip, either in advance or while you hike. Some people hike only 7 miles a day, while others happily cover more than 20; some hikers complete the entire trail in one go, while others hike a section at a time. This book caters to everyone: it provides information on distances along the trail, established camping locations, stretches of trail with steep ascents and descents, and lateral trails that access the JMT. From there, you design the itinerary that best suits you.

The introductory material provides information on three essential JMT topics: how to obtain a wilderness permit, how to get yourself to and from the two endpoints using either public transportation or a private shuttle, and how to arrange food resupplies along the trail. All of the phone numbers and websites required for your planning are supplied. Also provided are area maps of Yosemite Valley, Tuolumne Meadows, and Lone Pine to orient you at trailheads, as well as a map showing air and shuttle-bus transportation options that access the JMT.

Next are 16 topographic maps, onto which trail junctions and campsites (listed in the table beginning on page 64) have been plotted. These maps are derived from the latest digital elevation models available from the US Geological Survey. Overlaid on these are layers with information on water bodies, roads, and geographic names, also courtesy of the USGS. As for the trails, the JMT and all side trails shown are derived from GPS tracks that I have collected over the past decade. I hiked all of the trails shown while carrying two GPS units, each logging a data point every 6–8 seconds; I then plotted the resulting tracks on a satellite photo and further edited the tracks to precisely match the actual track. Distances in the book are derived from these tracks. See "Maps" (page 16) for additional information.

The topographic maps are followed by the trail data. Mirroring the organization of the larger JMT book, the trail information is split into 13 sections, one for each of the river drainages through which the JMT passes. Each section includes a detailed elevation profile of the trail and a table listing major waypoints, including most trail junctions. Each waypoint entry in the tables includes the elevation, GPS coordinates (expressed as latitude and longitude), the distance from the previous point, and the cumulative distance from the JMT's northern terminus, Happy Isles.

At the end of the book is some extra data. First is a table listing established, legal campsites. For each campsite, information provided includes the cumulative trail distance, the GPS coordinates, a brief description, and whether campfires are permitted. The next section comprises elevation profiles, data tables, and two maps for lateral trails feeding into the JMT—this information is valuable if you plan to section-hike the JMT, or if you unexpectedly have to exit the wilderness and need to determine the most efficient way to exit. The section on lateral trails is followed by a table listing emergency numbers for the jurisdictions through which the JMT passes and the locations of wilderness ranger stations.

I wish you a wonderful trip on the JMT. Enjoy the superb surroundings as you traipse along a trail that commemorates one of the world's most influential conservationists.

—Elizabeth Wenk

Planning Your Hike

Wilderness Permits

All trailheads accessing the JMT require a wilderness permit and have quotas. For all Sierra wilderness areas, permits are issued for the trailhead and date at which you begin your hike. You do not need to obtain a new permit after exiting the wilderness for a food resupply.

If you are getting a permit issued by **Inyo National Forest** and you plan to exit at **Trail Crest,** note that you are subject to the Mount Whitney exit quota, capped at 25 people per day. Likewise, just 45 hikers per day with authorized permits may leave **Yosemite National Park** at **Donohue Pass.** Donahue exit permits are issued in conjunction with two Yosemite wilderness permits: **Happy Isles–Past Little Yosemite Valley** and **Lyell Canyon Trailhead.**

A word of warning: Quotas for permits fill very quickly in summer. So reserve your permit as soon as they become available, and, if possible, choose alternative weekday start dates as potential backups.

Starting in 2022, reservable permits for all wilderness areas along the JMT are available through **Recreation.gov.** A benefit of using Recreation.gov is that you can easily see which days still have available permits, and you can also quickly note when permits become available due to cancellations.

Permit Reservation and Pickup Details

All agencies release permits not picked up by 10 a.m. the day of the permit (occasionally 9 a.m.), reallocating the permit to someone waiting for a first-come, first-served

---

PERMIT-RESERVATION INFORMATION

Yosemite NP • **When to Reserve** 24 weeks in advance, with weekly mini-lottery**
• **How to Reserve** Recreation.gov • **Cost** $5 per permit; + $5 per person; + $10 fee to enter the lottery
• **Percent of Permits Available for Reservation** 60%
• **First-Come, First-Served Permit Availability*** 11 a.m. day before entry

Inyo NF • **When to Reserve** 7 a.m. Pacific time, 6 months in advance • **How to Reserve** Recreation.gov
• **Cost** $6 per permit + $5 per person*** • **Percent of Permits Available for Reservation** 60%
• **First-Come, First-Served Permit Availability*** 11 a.m. day before entry, but request form can be filled in at 8 a.m.

Whitney Portal (Inyo NF) • **When to Reserve** Enter lottery February 1–March 15
• **How to Reserve** Recreation.gov • **Cost** $6 per reservation + $15 per person • **Percent of Permits Available for Reservation** 100% • **First-Come, First-Served Permit Availability** *only cancellations available

Sierra NF • **When to Reserve** 7 a.m. Pacific time, 6 months in advance • **How to Reserve** Recreation.gov
• **Cost** $6 per permit + $5 per person*** • **Percent of Permits Available for Reservation** 60%
• **First-Come, First-Served Permit Availability*** wilderness station opening, day before entry

Sequoia/Kings Canyon NP • **When to Reserve** 7 a.m. Pacific time, 6 months in advance
• **How to Reserve** Recreation.gov • **Cost** $15 per permit + $5 per person
• **Percent of Permits Available for Reservation** about 75%
• **First-Come, First-Served Permit Availability*** 1 p.m. day before entry

---

*   First-come, first-served permits have been dispensed online in 2020, 2021, and 2022 due to COVID-19, with most agencies releasing permits 1–2 weeks in advance of the permit date.
**   During any given Sunday–Saturday, reservations are submitted for a 1-week window 24 weeks later. At the end of the week, a mini-lottery is held. See nps.gov/yose/planyourvisit/wildpermitdates.htm for details.
*** $15 per person if exiting at Whitney Portal

permit. If you know you won't be able to pick up your permit by this time, call ahead and it will be held for you until you arrive.

Yosemite National Park Wilderness Permits
PERMIT RESERVATIONS: recreation.gov/permits/445859
WILDERNESS INFORMATION: 209-372-0826 (Monday–Friday, 9 a.m.–4:30 p.m.)
nps.gov/yose/planyourvisit/wildpermits.htm

Permits for **Happy Isles** can be picked up at the **Yosemite Valley Wilderness Center,** in Yosemite Village between the post office and the Ansel Adams Gallery. Permits for **Lyell Canyon** and other Tuolumne Meadows trailheads can be picked up at the **Tuolumne Meadows Wilderness Center,** along Tuolumne Meadows Lodge Road. See nps.gov/yose/planyourvisit/permitstations.htm for maps.

Inyo National Forest Wilderness Permits
PERMIT RESERVATIONS: recreation.gov/permits/233262 (permits for all trailheads except Whitney Portal); recreation.gov/permits/233260 (Whitney Portal permits)
WILDERNESS INFORMATION: 760-873-2483 (8 a.m.–4:30 p.m.; off-season, Monday–Friday; May 15–October 15, open every day)
fs.usda.gov/main/inyo/passes-permits/recreation

Permits can be picked up at one of four US Forest Service offices along the US 395 corridor:

Mono Basin Scenic Area Visitor Center (in northeastern Lee Vining)
1 Visitor Center Drive, Lee Vining, CA 9354; 760-647-3044
SUMMER HOURS: 8:30 a.m.–4:30 p.m.

Mammoth Lakes Welcome Center
2510 Main St., Mammoth Lakes, CA 93546; 760-924-5500
SUMMER HOURS: 9 a.m.–5 p.m.

White Mountain Public Lands Information Center (in Bishop)
798 N. Main St., Bishop, CA 93514; 760-873-2500
SUMMER HOURS: 8:30 a.m.–4:30 p.m.

Eastern Sierra Visitor Center (in Lone Pine)
Junction of US 395 and CA 136, 2 miles south of Lone Pine; 760-876-6200
SUMMER HOURS: 8 a.m.–4:30 p.m.

Permits for trips entering one of the three national parks—**Yosemite, Sequoia,** and **Kings Canyon**—must be picked up in person; if your trip remains entirely on national-forest lands, you can call in advance and request that your permit be left in a drop box.

Sierra National Forest Wilderness Permits
PERMIT RESERVATIONS: recreation.gov/permits/445858
WILDERNESS INFORMATION: 559-855-5355, ext. 3301 (Prather office: 8 a.m.–4:30 p.m.; off-season, Monday–Friday; June–September, open every day)
tinyurl.com/sierrapermit, tinyurl.com/sierrawilderness

Permits can be picked up at the main **High Sierra Ranger District Office** (29688 Auberry Road, Prather, CA 93651) or at the **High Sierra Visitor Information Station,** 15.7 miles along Kaiser Pass Road. If you call the Prather office in advance, someone will leave your permit in a drop box.

Sequoia and Kings Canyon National Parks Wilderness Permits
PERMIT RESERVATIONS: recreation.gov/permits/445857
WILDERNESS INFORMATION: 559-565-3766
nps.gov/seki/planyourvisit/wilderness_permits.htm

Permits for the **Woods Creek** and **Bubbs Creek Trailheads** must be picked up in person at the **Roads End Permit Station,** open 7 a.m.–3:30 p.m. daily. The permit station is located at the far eastern end of Kings Canyon, aka the Roads End. Check the Sequoia and Kings Canyon National Parks website (above) if you are entering from a different trailhead.

Transportation

There are two distinct transportation challenges you face while hiking the JMT: how to get to (and from) the Sierra and how to get back to your car at the end of your trip. This section outlines your transportation options.

People living outside of California will probably begin their journey to a JMT trailhead on a plane. Transportation to the Sierra is available from airports in the San Francisco Bay Area and Los Angeles International Airport (LAX), as well as from smaller airports, including Mammoth Lakes, Reno, and Merced. See "Routes to and from the Sierra" (page 7) for public transit connections to and from these airports, which are listed in order of size, from bigger (and farther from the Sierra) to smaller (and generally closer to the Sierra).

Yosemite Area Regional Transportation System (**YARTS**) buses deliver you close to trailheads in Yosemite Valley and Tuolumne Meadows. For trailheads in the Mammoth Lakes region, you can take YARTS or **Eastern Sierra Transit** (**EST**) buses to the town and then take local EST-run bus services or the Devils Postpile/Reds Meadow bus to the trailheads. To reach trailheads not accessible by public transport, a selection of charter services is available (see page 8). See the table in "Lateral Trails" (pages 84–87) for additional trail information; also see the map on the next page.

Transit-Agency Contact Information

AGENCY	TYPE	WEBSITE	PHONE
Amtrak	train and bus	amtrak.com	800-USA-RAIL (800-872-7245) or 215-856-7924
Antelope Valley Airport Express	bus	antelopeexpress.com	661-947-2529
BART (Bay Area Rapid Transit)	commuter rail	bart.gov	510-465-2278
Eastern Sierra Transit Authority (ESTA)	bus	estransit.com	800-922-1930; or 760-872-1901 (Bishop) 760-924-3184 (Mammoth Lakes) 760-614-0030 (Lone Pine)
YARTS (Yosemite Area Regional Transit System)	bus	yarts.com	877-989-2787
Aramark (Yosemite Concessionaire)	bus	travelyosemite.com /things-to-do/guided -bus-tours	888-413-8869
Sequoia Shuttle*	bus	sequoiashuttle.com	877-BUS-HIKE (287-4453)

*This is of limited utility to JMT hikers but can be used by hikers joining the High Sierra Trail and the JMT.

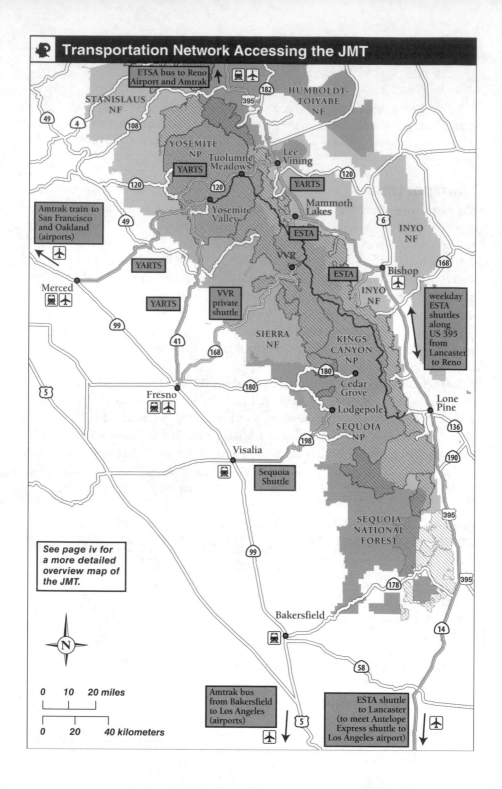

Transportation Network Accessing the JMT

STANISLAUS NF

HUMBOLDT-TOIYABE NF

ETSA bus to Reno Airport and Amtrak

YOSEMITE NP

Tuolumne Meadows

YARTS

Lee Vining

YARTS

Mammoth Lakes

Yosemite Valley

ESTA

VVR

Amtrak train to San Francisco and Oakland (airports)

YARTS

Bishop

INYO NF

ESTA

weekday ESTA shuttles along US 395 from Lancaster to Reno

Merced

YARTS

VVR private shuttle

INYO NF

SIERRA NF

KINGS CANYON NP

Fresno

Cedar Grove

Lodgepole

Lone Pine

Visalia

SEQUOIA NP

Sequoia Shuttle

See page iv for a more detailed overview map of the JMT.

SEQUOIA NATIONAL FOREST

N

0   10   20 miles

0   20   40 kilometers

Bakersfield

Amtrak bus from Bakersfield to Los Angeles (airports)

ESTA shuttle to Lancaster (to meet Antelope Express shuttle to Los Angeles airport)

Transit Route Information
ROUTES TO AND FROM THE SIERRA

ROUTE	AGENCY (Route)	TRIP DURATION (Hours)	TRIP FREQUENCY
SFO or OAK ↔ Richmond	BART	1	Every 20–30 minutes
SFO ↔ Embarcadero (SF CBD)	BART	0.5	Every 20–30 minutes
Embarcadero (SF CBD) ↔ Emeryville	Amtrak (bus)	0.5	Timed to meet each train to/from Merced or Reno
Richmond or Emeryville ↔ Merced	Amtrak (train)	3	5 times daily
Richmond or Emeryville ↔ Reno	Amtrak (train or train/bus)	5–6.5	Twice daily
Merced Amtrak station ↔ Yosemite Valley	YARTS (Blue route)	3	5–6 times daily
Fresno airport/Amtrak station ↔ Yosemite Valley	YARTS (Yellow route)	3.5	3 times daily, May 10–September 10
Reno ↔ Mammoth Lakes ↔ Lone Pine	ESTA (US 395 Northbound)	6	Once daily, Monday–Friday; no weekend service
Lancaster ↔ Lone Pine ↔ Mammoth Lakes	ESTA (US 395 Southbound)	5	Once daily, Monday–Friday; no weekend service
LAX ↔ Lancaster	Antelope Express	2	8 times daily
Los Angeles ↔ Fresno	Amtrak (train/bus)	5–5.5	6 times daily

ROUTES BETWEEN SIERRA TOWNS AND TO TRAILHEADS

ROUTE	AGENCY (Route)	TRIP DURATION (Hours)	TRIP FREQUENCY
Mammoth Lakes ↔ Tuolumne Meadows ↔ Yosemite Valley	YARTS (Green route)	4	Twice daily, July, August; once daily, June 15–July 1, September 1–October 15 (north-, then westbound trips in the morning; east-, then southbound trips in the afternoon)
Tuolumne Meadows ↔ Yosemite Valley	Aramark (Yosemite Valley to Tuolumne Meadows Hikers Bus)	3	Once daily
Bishop ↔ Lone Pine	ESTA (Lone Pine Express)	1	4 times daily, Monday–Friday; no weekend service
Bishop ↔ Mammoth Lakes	ESTA (Mammoth Express)	1	4 times daily, Monday–Friday; no weekend service
Tuolumne Meadows shuttle (Tenaya Lake ↔ Tuolumne Meadows locations)	Aramark (Yosemite concessionaire)	0.5	Every 30 minutes, July–early September
Mammoth Lakes ↔ Reds Meadow, Devils Postpile, Agnew Meadows Trailheads	ESTA (Reds Meadow Shuttle)	1	Every 20–30 minutes, July–mid-September
Mammoth Lakes ↔ Red Cones Trailhead, Duck Pass Trailhead	ESTA (Lakes Basin Trolley)	1	Every 30 minutes, July–early September
Bishop ↔ South Lake, North Lake, Lake Sabrina Trailheads	ESTA (Bishop Creek Shuttle)	1	Twice daily, mid-June–early September
Fresno ↔ Vermilion Valley Resort (VVR), Florence Lake	VVR Trailhead Shuttle*	3–4+	Once daily
Visalia ↔ Lodgepole	Sequoia Shuttle	See right	Call 877-287-4453 for schedule details

*This is a scheduled private van service run by VVR; see edisonlake.com/hikers/transportation.

Car Rental Agencies

Enterprise
85 Airport Road, Mammoth Lakes, CA 93546
909-204-1759
187 W. Line St., Bishop, CA 93514
760-873-3704; enterprise.com

National
85 Airport Road, Mammoth Lakes, CA 93546
909-204-1759; national.com

Charter Services

The businesses and individuals listed below are licensed to provide private shuttles between trailheads.

Lone Pine Chamber of Commerce
760-876-4444 or 208-863-6975
lonepinechamber.org/services-available-chamber-of-commerce

Mt. Williamson Motel and Basecamp (based in Independence)
760-878-2121
mtwilliamsonmotel.com; info@mtwilliamsonmotel.com
(*Note:* Provides shuttle services for paying motel guests only.)

East Side Sierra Shuttle (Paul Fretheim; based in Independence)
760-878-8047
eastsidesierrashuttle.com; paul@inyopro.com

Sierra Shuttle Service (Robert Brence; based in Mammoth Lakes)
760-914-2746
sierrashuttleservice.com; sierrashuttleservices@outlook.com

Mammoth All Weather Shuttle (MAWS)
760-709-2927
mawshuttle.com/about-us

Mammoth Taxi
760-937-8294
mammoth-taxi.com

Trailhead Maps

Maps of **Yosemite Valley** (page 10), **Tuolumne Meadows** (page 11), and **Lone Pine** (page 12) will help orient you at the main trailheads.

Food Resupplies

In general, you have three options for replenishing your food supply along the trail. You can exit the trail to pick up food at a resort, post office, or one of the package-holding services listed on page 15; have a friend or a courier service (page 15) drive your food to a trailhead; or have your food packed into the JMT by stock.

LOCATION	DISTANCE FROM HAPPY ISLES	DISTANCE FROM WHITNEY PORTAL	TYPE OF RESUPPLY	DISTANCE TO RESUPPLY/TRAILHEAD FROM JMT
Tuolumne Meadows	22.7 miles	199.5	post office/trailhead food-storage lockers	0.25 miles
Red's Meadow Resort/ Mammoth Lakes	59.4 miles	162.8	resort/post office	0.25 miles (resort)
NOTES: additional 1-hour shuttle ride to Mammoth Lakes Post Office or stores in Mammoth Lakes				
Vermilion Valley Resort (VVR)	88.2 miles	134.0	resort	6.8 miles (no ferry); 1.5 miles (with ferry)
NOTES: The table on page 81 describes 4 alternate trails to VVR: Goodale Pass, Lake Edison Trail, Bear Ridge Trail, and Bear Creek Trail.				
Muir Trail Ranch (MTR)	108.5 miles	111.9	resort	0.25 miles
Bishop Pass	137.8 miles	84.4	resort/post office/stock resupply	12.4 miles
NOTES: additional 1.3 miles down road to Parchers Resort or 22 miles to post office, stores, and hiker hostel in Bishop; twice-daily shuttle to Bishop				
Woods Creek	169.6 miles	52.6	stock resupply	0.0 miles
Kearsarge Pass	180.6 miles	41.6	hiker hostel/post office/stock resupply/ trailhead food-storage lockers	7.7 miles
NOTES: additional 13 miles down road to post office and hiker hostel in Independence				

Key resupply locations are listed in the table above and in the section below; also see the list of post offices starting on page 12 for additional, less frequently used options. Each resupply location has its own suggestions for how long in advance you should send packages, but in general, you should aim to have your resupply package arrive 2–3 weeks before you do, due to the remoteness of some resorts.

Also see page 7 for a summary of the public shuttle options from trailheads.

Three Most Commonly Used Resorts

Red's Meadow Resort (redsmeadow.com) Accessed from either the eastern or western Reds Meadow junctions or from Devils Postpile. See the Devils Postpile map on page 13 for trails in the area.

Vermilion Valley Resort (edisonlake.com; vermilionvalley.com) Accessed from the Lake Edison Trail, Lake Edison Ferry, Goodale Pass Trail, Bear Ridge Trail, or Bear Creek Trail. The Lake Edison Ferry costs $28 round-trip. It usually runs twice daily, leaving the VVR landing at 9 a.m. and 4 p.m., and leaving the ferry wharf on the east side of Lake Edison at 9:45 a.m. and 4:45 p.m. See page 81 for additional information on how best to access VVR, and see pages 82–83 for a map of the area.

Muir Trail Ranch (muirtrailranch.com) Accessed from either the northern or southern Muir Trail Ranch cutoff. The ranch is on a spur trail along the trail to Florence Lake.

(continued on page 12)

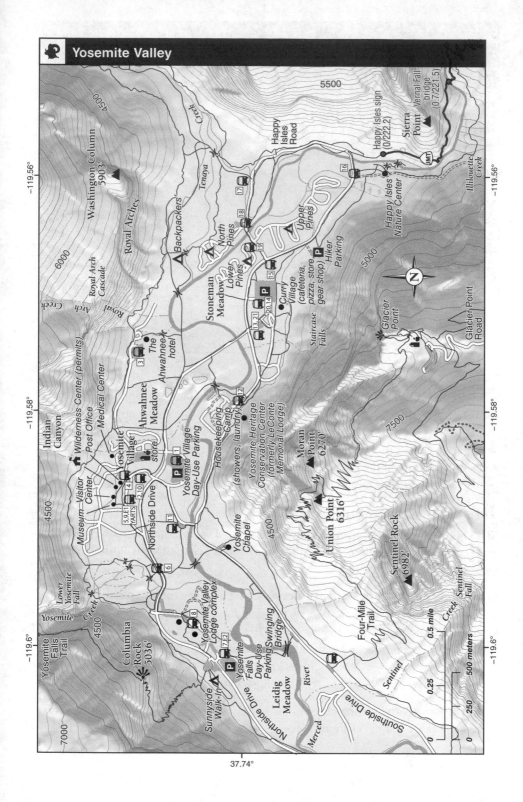

Vernal Fall
bridge
(0.7/221.5)

5500

Happy Isles sign
(0/222.2)

Sierra
Point

Happy Isles
Road

Illilouette
Creek

JMT

Happy Isles
Nature Center

Washington
Column
5903'

Royal Arches

Backpackers'

Tenaya

Creek

17

18

North
Pines

Upper
Pines

5000

19

Glacier
Point

6000

Royal
Arch
Cascade

Lower
Pines

15

Stoneman
Meadow

Curry
Village
(cafeteria,
pizza, store,
gear shop)

Hiker
Parking

Staircase
Falls

Glacier
Point
Road

Royal
Arch
Creek

20,14

13, 21

5000

7500

The
Ahwahnee
hotel

3

Indian
Canyon

Wilderness Center (permits)
Post Office
Medical Center

Ahwahnee
Meadow

12

Yosemite Heritage
Conservation Center
(formerly LeConte
Memorial Lodge)

Moran
Point
6270'

Housekeeping
Camp
(showers, laundry)

Yosemite
Village

store

1

Museum–Visitor
Center

Yosemite Village
Day-Use Parking

Union Point
6316'

4500

4500

4

2,10

5,9,E1

YARTS

Northside Drive

1

Yosemite
Chapel

Sentinel Rock
6982'

6

Lower Yosemite
Fall

Yosemite
Falls
Trail

4500

Columbia
Rock
5036'

8

Yosemite Valley
Lodge complex

7,2

Yosemite
Falls
Day-Use
Parking

Swinging
Bridge

Four-Mile
Trail

Sentinel
Fall

7000

Yosemite

Creek

Sunnyside
Walk-In

Leidig
Meadow

Northside Drive

Southside Drive

Sentinel
Creek

Merced
River

0.5 mile

0.25

500 meters

250

0

37.74°

−119.56°

−119.58°

−119.6°

−119.56°

−119.58°

−119.6°

Z

10

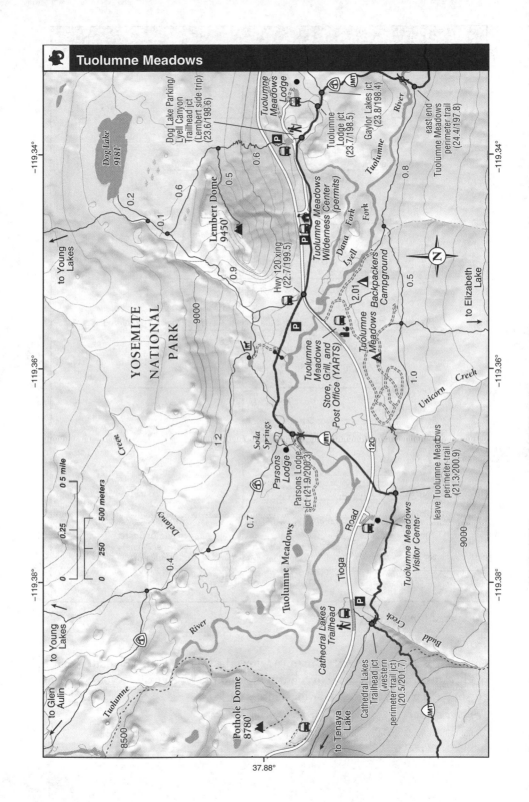

YOSEMITE NATIONAL PARK

Dog Lake
9181'

Lembert Dome
9450'

Dog Lake Parking/
Lyell Canyon
Trailhead jct
(Lembert side trip)
(23.6/198.6)

Tuolumne
Lodge

Tuolumne
Meadows

Tuolumne
Lodge jct
(23.7/198.5)

Gaylor Lakes jct
(23.8/198.4)

east end
Tuolumne Meadows
perimeter trail
(24.4/197.8)

Tuolumne Meadows
Wilderness Center
(permits)

Hwy 120 xing
(22.7/199.5)

Dana Fork

Lyell Fork

Tuolumne River

Tuolumne Meadows
Backpackers'
Campground

2.0!

to Elizabeth
Lake

Unicorn Creek

to Young
Lakes

9000

Tuolumne Meadows
Store, Grill, and
Post Office (YARTS)

Soda
Springs

Parsons
Lodge

Parsons Lodge
jct (21.9/200.3)

1.2

1.0

leave Tuolumne Meadows
perimeter trail
(21.3/200.9)

Tuolumne Meadows
Visitor Center

9000

Delaney Creek

Tuolumne Meadows

0.7

Tioga Road

Cathedral Lakes
Trailhead

to Young
Lakes

River

0.4

to Glen
Aulin

Tuolumne

Pothole Dome
8780'

8500

Cathedral Lakes
Trailhead jct
(western
perimeter trail jct)
(20.5/201.7)

Budd Creek

to Tenaya
Lake

0 0.5 mile

0 0.25

0 250 500 meters

11

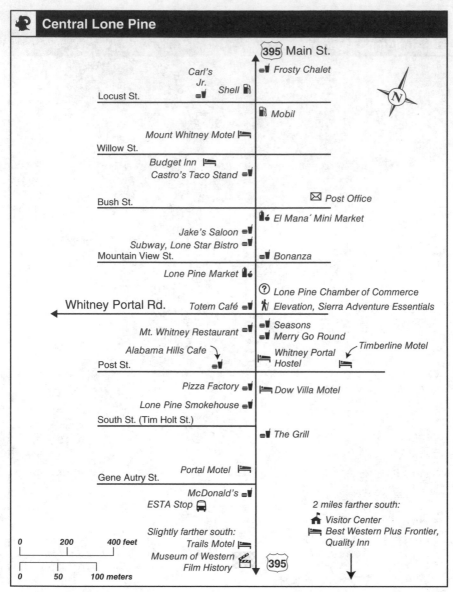

(continued from page 9)

Post Offices

Following is a list of post offices in towns along the JMT, in north-to-south order; call or check usps.com in advance to confirm their hours. When mailing your package to any of these places, use the following address:

[your name]
c/o General Delivery
[name of post office]
[address]
[city], CA [zip code]
Hold until [date]

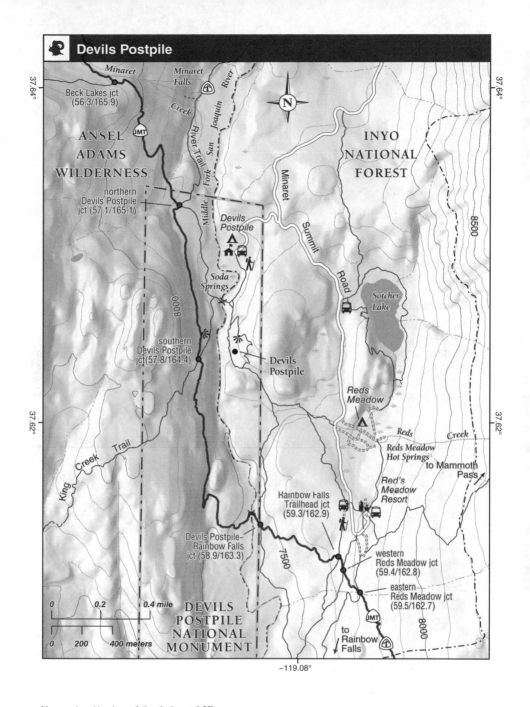

Yosemite National Park Post Office
9017 Village Drive
Yosemite National Park, CA 95389-9998; 209-372-4475
NEARBY SERVICES: general store, restaurants, camping, outdoor-gear shop
HOURS: Monday–Friday, 8:30 a.m.–5 p.m.; Sat, 10 a.m.–noon

(continued on next page)

Tuolumne Meadows Post Office
14000 CA 120 E.
Yosemite National Park, CA 95389-9906; 209-372-8236
NEARBY SERVICES: general store with fuel, restaurant, camping
HOURS: Monday–Friday, 9 a.m.–5 p.m.; Sat, 9 a.m.–noon

Lee Vining Post Office
121 Lee Vining Ave.
Lee Vining, CA 93541-9997; 760-647-6371
NEARBY SERVICES: hotels, restaurants, general store with fuel, USFS office, camping
HOURS: Monday–Friday, 9 a.m.–4 p.m. (closed 1 p.m.–2 p.m. for lunch)

June Lake Post Office
2747 Boulder Drive
June Lake, CA 93529-9997; 760-648-7483
NEARBY SERVICES: hotels, restaurants, general store, camping
HOURS: Monday–Friday, 8 a.m.–3 p.m. (closed 12:30 p.m.–1 p.m. for lunch)

Mammoth Lakes Post Office
3330 Main St.
Mammoth Lakes, CA 93546-9997; 760-934-2205
NEARBY SERVICES: hotels, restaurants, outdoor gear shops, food stores, USFS, camping
HOURS: Monday–Friday, 8 a.m.–4 p.m.

Bishop Post Office
585 W. Line St.
Bishop, CA 93514-9998; 760-873-3526
NEARBY SERVICES: hiker hostel, hotels, restaurants, outdoor gear shops, food stores, USFS office, camping
HOURS: Monday–Friday, 9 a.m.–4 p.m.; Sat, 9 a.m.–1 p.m.

Independence Post Office
101 S. Edwards St.
Independence, CA 93526-9997; 760-878-2210
NEARBY SERVICES: hiker hostel, hotels, restaurants
HOURS: Monday–Friday, 9:30 a.m.–4 p.m., (closed 12:45 p.m.–1:15 p.m. for lunch)

Lone Pine Post Office
121 E. Bush St.
Lone Pine, CA 93545-9997; 760-876-5681
NEARBY SERVICES: hotels, restaurants, outdoor gear shops, general store, USFS office
HOURS: Monday–Friday, 9:30 a.m.–4:30 p.m. (closed 12:30 p.m.–1:30 p.m. for lunch)

Mono Hot Springs Post Office
72000 CA 168
Mono Hot Springs, CA 93642-9800; 559-325-1710
NEARBY SERVICES: general store, fuel, restaurant, camping, hot springs; visit monohotsprings.com/post-office for more information.
HOURS: M–Sat, 9 a.m.–6 p.m.

Courier, Package-Holding, and Pack-Stock Services

A number of individuals and businesses simplify your food resupplies by allowing you to mail your food to them or by picking up your package from the post office; they will then hold it for you to pick up outside of post office hours. In addition, three of the services below use pack animals to bring your food to you. From north to south:

Parchers Resort
5001 S. Lake Road
Bishop, CA 93514
760-873-4177
parchersresort.net/backpackerservices.htm; info@parchersresort.net

Rainbow Pack Outfitters (Greg and Ruby Allen)
PO Box 1791
Bishop, CA 93515; 760-873-8877
rainbowpackoutfitters.com, info@rainbowpackoutfitters.com

Mt. Williamson Motel and Basecamp
PO Box 128
515 S. Edwards St. (US 395)
Independence, CA 93526
760-878-2121
mtwilliamsonmotel.com

Sequoia Kings Pack Trains (Brian and Danica Berner)
PO Box 209
Independence, CA 93526
800-962-0775 or 760-387-2797 (Danica)
bernerspack@yahoo.com

Cedar Grove Pack Station (Tim Loverin and Family)
108300 Cedar Lane
Kings Canyon National Park, CA 93633
559-565-3464 (summer); 559-802-7626 (winter)
cedargrovepackstation.com

Water Availability

Along the JMT, water is rarely more than a 5-minute walk from the trail. The exceptions are the upper sections of passes, which rarely contain watercourses, and occasional stretches of trail that traverse a slope. Later in the season, side creeks become sparser, as they are more likely to dry up, but along the JMT the only rivers marked as permanent that I have seen vanish are around Sunrise High Sierra Camp (mile 13.0), the outlet of Trinity Creek (mile 53.9), the upper stretches of Silver Pass Creek (miles 83.8–84.7), and the waterways around Sandy Meadow (miles 201.7–202.6). As well as the major streams, springs tend to be reliable late in the season and are often indicated on maps.

The abundance of water sources means that unless you wish to camp high (for example, on the summit of Mount Whitney) or dry (to avoid bugs), you can mostly carry a single quart (liter) of water at a time, filling up with 2 quarts (2 liters) over passes and for the sections of trail detailed below. I advocate always carrying a liter of water; running out of water for even a short stretch puts you at severe risk of dehydration.

The stretches of trail that last longer than 2.5 miles without any water, or with few opportunities to refill, are listed in the table below.

Starting Mileage	Starting Location	Ending Mileage	Ending Location	Distance Without Water	Notes
0.7	Vernal Fall bridge	3.1	top Nevada Fall	2.4 miles	—
10.3	Sunrise Creek	17.1	Upper Cathedral Lake	6.8 miles	water almost always available at Sunrise backpackers' camp
45.5	Garnet Lake outlet	48.5	Shadow Creek	3.0 miles	—
51.6	Gladys Lake	56.1	Minaret Creek	4.5 miles	pass Trinity Lakes at a distance
56.1	Minaret Creek	58.8	Middle Fork San Joaquin River	2.7 miles	—
65.2	Deer Creek	70.4	Duck Creek	5.2 miles	
80.9	Chief Lake	85.4	Mott Lake junction	4.5 miles	Silver Pass Lake has water; usually some in Silver Pass Creek
88.5	just south of Mono Creek	94.6	near Bear Creek	6.1 miles	small creek on north side; spring on south side usually reliable
106.4	Senger Creek	112.1	Piute Creek	5.7 miles	water at Muir Trail Ranch; spring near northern MTR cutoff junction usually reliable
145.7	base Golden Staircase	147.6	top Golden Staircase	1.9 miles	short distance, but hot and exposed; difficult to reach creek
149.6	above Upper Palisade Lake	153.6	Upper Basin	4.0 miles	—
200.4	Wallace Creek tributary	204.1	Crabtree Meadow camping area	3.7 miles	—
206.8	Guitar Lake	216.0	Trail Camp	9.2 miles	—

Maps

This book includes maps for the JMT and some of the trailheads; they show the way-points and mileages listed in the tables for each of the 13 trail sections. These maps are perfectly adequate for following the trail, knowing the mileage you have walked, and turning in the correct direction at each junction. If you wish to supplement them with paper maps, **Tom Harrison** (tom harrisonmaps.com) and *National Geographic* Trails Illustrated (natgeomaps.com) maps are popular.

A GPS-uploadable file with all of the waypoints in this guidebook is available at tinyurl .com/JMTWaypoints.

Meanwhile, more and more hikers are ditching paper maps in favor of digital ones. Of these, the app **Gaia GPS** (gaiagps.com) is the most widely used and allows you to upload both waypoints (that is, those provided in this book) and USGS 7.5-minute topo maps. **CalTopo** (caltopo.com) offers a similar service. That said, if you rely on apps alone, you'll miss out on that wonderful sense of connectedness to the entire landscape that you'll have if you look at your trip on a giant mosaic of paper maps.

One option, for either paper or digital maps, is to take advantage of online services that let you plot out routes and make plans in advance of your trip, then to print out your own maps at the exact scale you want. If you print on Rite in the Rain paper (sold by the sheet), your maps will last the duration of your trip. Look at these websites for good map interfaces:

CalTopo (caltopo.com/about) is a website and mobile app for making custom maps.

US Geological Survey TopoView (tinyurl.com/mapstopo) hosts all USGS topographic maps, including historical maps. The URL above focuses on the Yosemite area. *Note:* The available maps won't appear until you click on the screen.

The National Map (apps.nationalmap.gov/viewer) is an online USGS map interface.

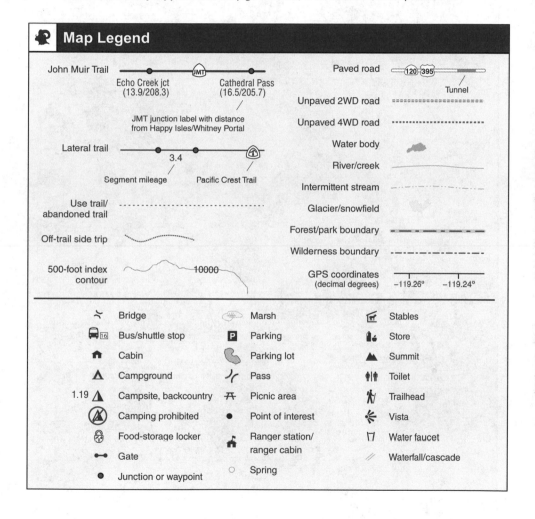

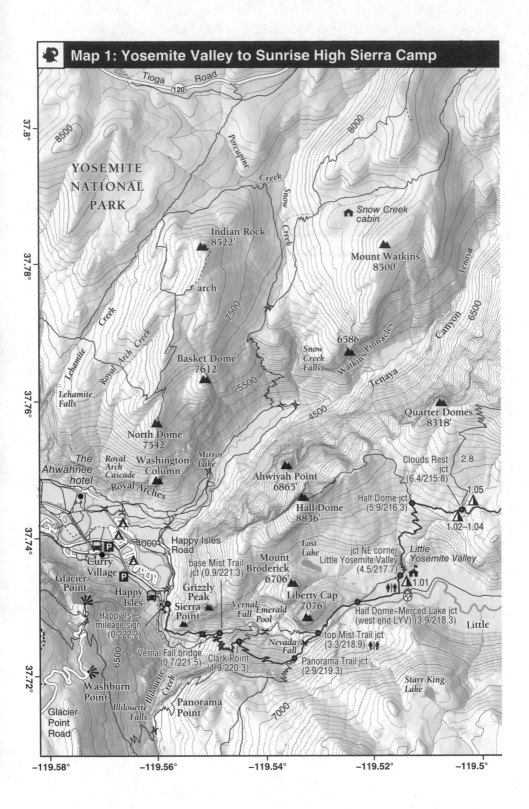

Tioga Road
120

YOSEMITE NATIONAL PARK

8500

Porcupine

Creek

8000

Snow Creek cabin

Snow Creek

Indian Rock 8522'

Mount Watkins 8500'

Tenaya

arch

7500

6586'

Snow Creek Falls

Watkins Pinnacles

6500

Lehamite Creek

Royal Arch Creek

Basket Dome 7612'

5500

Tenaya Canyon

Quarter Domes 8318'

Lehamite Falls

North Dome 7542'

4500

Clouds Rest jct (6.4/215.8)

2.8

Royal Arch Cascade

Washington Column

Mirror Lake

Ahwiyah Point 6865'

Half Dome jct (5.9/216.3)

1.05

The Ahwahnee hotel

Royal Arches

Half Dome 8836'

1.02–1.04

Happy Isles Road

Lost Lake

jct NE corner Little Yosemite Valley (4.5/217.7)

Little Yosemite Valley

4000

base Mist Trail jct (0.9/221.3)

Mount Broderick 6706'

Curry Village

P

P

Glacier Point

Happy Isles

Grizzly Peak Sierra Point

Vernal Fall

Emerald Pool

Liberty Cap 7076'

1.01

Happy Isles mileage sign (0/222.2)

Nevada Fall

Half Dome–Merced Lake jct (west end LYV) (3.9/218.3)

Little

6500

Vernal Fall bridge (0.7/221.5)

Clark Point (1.9/220.3)

top Mist Trail jct (3.3/218.9)

Washburn Point

Illilouette Creek

Panorama Trail jct (2.9/219.3)

Starr King Lake

Glacier Point Road

Illilouette Falls

Panorama Point

7000

37.8°
37.78°
37.76°
37.74°
37.72°

−119.58° −119.56° −119.54° −119.52° −119.5°

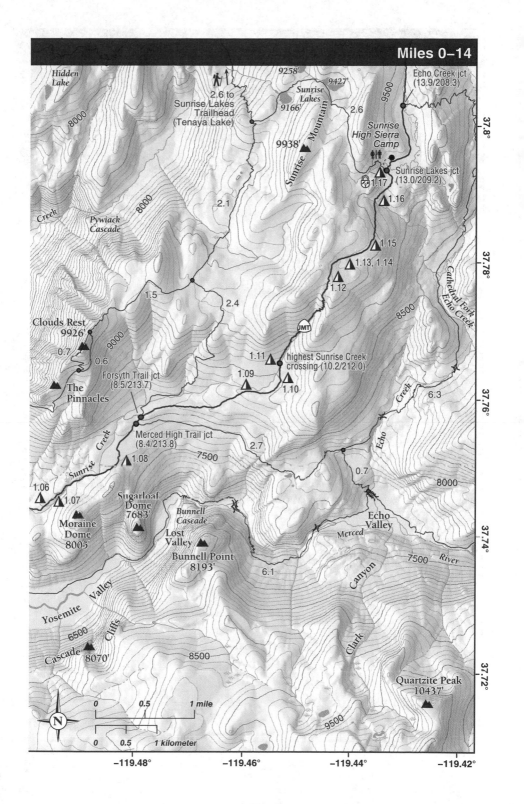

Hidden Lake

9258'

Echo Creek jct
(13.9/208.3)

Sunrise Lakes
9427'

2.6 to
Sunrise Lakes
Trailhead
(Tenaya Lake)

9166'

Sunrise
High Sierra
Camp

2.6

37.8°

9500

9938'

Sunrise Mountain

Sunrise Lakes jct
(13.0/209.2)

1.17

1.16

Creek

Pywiack
Cascade

8000

8000

2.1

1.15

1.13, 1.14

1.12

37.78°

2.4

1.5

Clouds Rest
9926'

9000

0.7

0.6

UMT

highest Sunrise Creek
crossing (10.2/212.0)

1.11

8500

Cathedral Fork Echo Creek

37.76°

Forsyth Trail jct
(8.5/213.7)

The
Pinnacles

1.09

1.10

6.3

Echo Creek

Merced High Trail jct
(8.4/213.8)

1.08

Sunrise Creek

7500

2.7

0.7

8000

1.06

1.07

Sugarloaf
Dome
7683'

Moraine
Dome
8005'

Bunnell
Cascade

Lost
Valley

Bunnell Point
8193'

6.1

Echo
Valley

Merced

River

7500

Yosemite Valley

Cliffs

Cascade
8070'

6500

8500

Clark Canyon

9500

Quartzite Peak
10437'

37.74°

37.72°

0   0.5   1 mile

N

0   0.5   1 kilometer

−119.48°   −119.46°   −119.44°   −119.42°

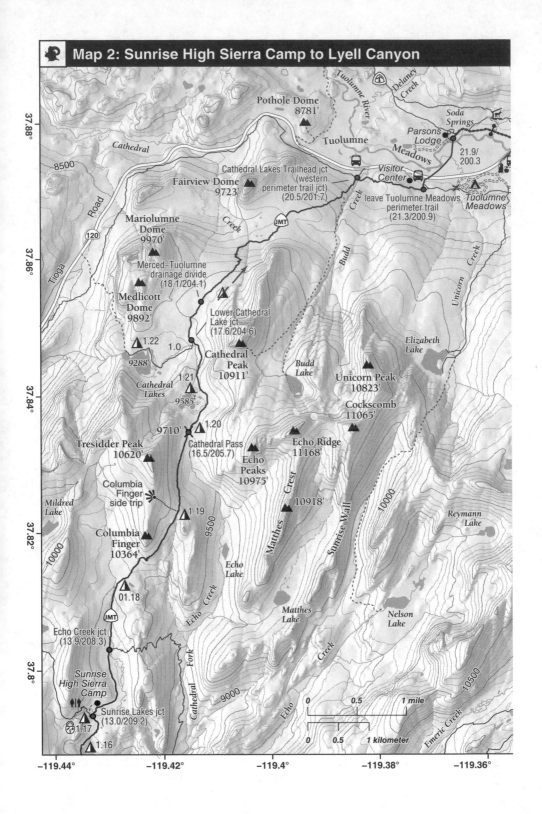

Delaney Creek

Tuolumne River

Soda Springs

Pothole Dome 8781'

Parsons Lodge

Tuolumne

21.9/ 200.3

Cathedral

8500

Cathedral Lakes Trailhead jct (western perimeter trail jct) (20.5/201.7)

Visitor Center

Fairview Dome 9723'

leave Tuolumne Meadows perimeter trail (21.3/200.9)

Tuolumne Meadows

Road

JMT

Creek

Budd

Unicorn Creek

Tioga

120

Mariolumne Dome 9970'

Merced–Tuolumne drainage divide (18.1/204.1)

Elizabeth Lake

Medlicott Dome 9892'

1.22

1.0

Lower Cathedral Lake jct (17.6/204.6)

Budd Lake

Unicorn Peak 10823'

9288'

Cathedral Lakes

Cathedral Peak 10911'

Cockscomb 11065'

1.21

9585'

1.20

Echo Ridge 11168'

Tresidder Peak 10620'

9710'

Cathedral Pass (16.5/205.7)

Echo Peaks 10975'

Mildred Lake

Columbia Finger side trip

Matthes Crest

10918'

Sunrise Wall

10000

Reymann Lake

Columbia Finger 10364'

1.19

Echo Lake

10000

01.18

Echo Creek

9500

Matthes Lake

Nelson Lake

JMT

Echo Creek jct (13.9/208.3)

10500

Sunrise High Sierra Camp

Cathedral Fork

9000

Echo Creek

0   0.5   1 mile

Sunrise Lakes jct (13.0/209.2)

1.17

0   0.5   1 kilometer

Emeric Creek

1.16

37.88° 37.86° 37.84° 37.82° 37.8°

-119.44°   -119.42°   -119.4°   -119.38°   -119.36°

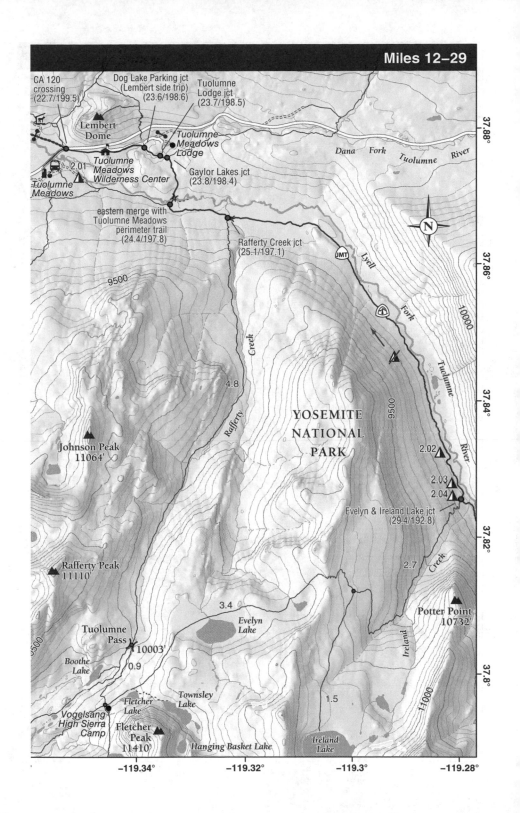

CA 120 crossing (22.7/199.5)

Dog Lake Parking jct (Lembert side trip) (23.6/198.6)

Tuolumne Lodge jct (23.7/198.5)

Lembert Dome

Tuolumne Meadows Lodge

2.01

Tuolumne Meadows Wilderness Center

Tuolumne Meadows

Gaylor Lakes jct (23.8/198.4)

Dana Fork Tuolumne River

eastern merge with Tuolumne Meadows perimeter trail (24.4/197.8)

Rafferty Creek jct (25.1/197.1)

N

JMT

Lyell

Fork

9500

4.8

Creek

10000

Tuolumne

9500

Rafferty

Johnson Peak 11064'

YOSEMITE NATIONAL PARK

River

2.02

2.03
2.04

Evelyn & Ireland Lake jct (29.4/192.8)

Rafferty Peak 11110'

2.7

Creek

Potter Point 10732'

3.4

Evelyn Lake

Ireland

9500

Tuolumne Pass

10003'

0.9

Boothe Lake

Townsley Lake

1.5

11000

Fletcher Lake

Vogelsang High Sierra Camp

Fletcher Peak 11410'

Hanging Basket Lake

Ireland Lake

−119.34°   −119.32°   −119.3°   −119.28°

37.88°

37.86°

37.84°

37.82°

37.8°

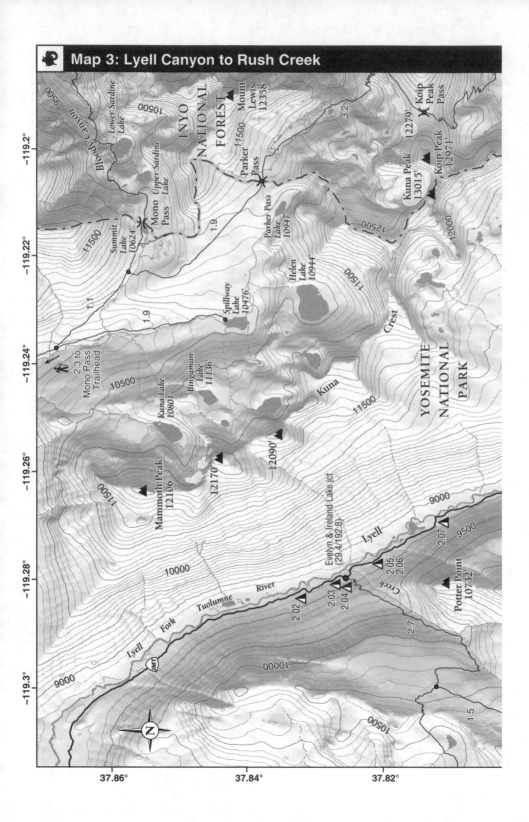

Blood Canyon 9500

Lower Sardine Lake

10500

INYO

NATIONAL FOREST

11,500'

Mount Lewis 12358'

3.2

Koip Peak Pass

Kuna Peak 12279'

Upper Sardine Lake

Mono Pass

Parker Pass

Koip Peak 12971'

Kuna Peak 13015'

11500

Summit Lake 10624'

Parker Pass

1.9

Parker Pass Lake 10947

12500

12000

1.1

1.9

Spillway Lake 10476'

Helen Lake 10944

11500

Crest

YOSEMITE

NATIONAL

PARK

2.3 to Mono Pass Trailhead

10500

Bingaman Lake 11136'

Kuna Lake 10801'

Kuna

11500

9000

Mammoth Peak 12106

12170'

12090'

Evelyn & Ireland Lake jct (29.4/192.8)

Lyell

2.07

9500

11500

10000

River

Tuolumne

Fork

Lyell

2.02

2.03

2.04

2.05, 2.06

Creek

Potter Point 10732'

9000

JMT

2.7

10000

9000

1.5

10500

N

37.86°   37.84°   37.82°

−119.2°
−119.22°
−119.24°
−119.26°
−119.28°
−119.3°

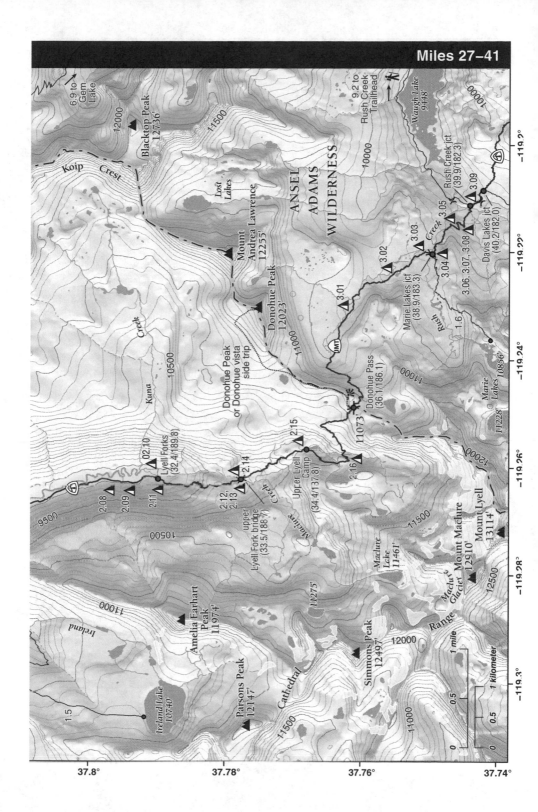

6.9 to Gem Lake

12000

Blacktop Peak 12736'

Koip Crest

11500

Lost Lakes

Mount Andrea Lawrence 12255'

Donohue Peak 12023'

Donohue Peak or Donohue vista side trip

ANSEL ADAMS WILDERNESS

9.2 to Rush Creek Trailhead

Waugh Lake 9448'

10000

Rush Creek Jct (39.9/182.3)

3.09

Davis Lakes jct (40.2/182.0)

3.05

3.03

Creek

3.02

3.04

3.06, 3.07, 3.08

Marie Lakes jct (38.9/183.3)

3.01

Rush

1.6

10000

10500

Creek

Kuna

10000

11000

JMT

Donohue Pass (36.1/186.1)

11073'

Marie Lakes 10856'

11000

11228

12000

12000

02.10

Lyell Forks (32.4/189.8)

2.15

Upper Lyell Camp (34.4/137.8)

2.16

2.08

2.09

2.11

9500

2.12, 2.13

2.14

Lyell Fork upper bridge (33.5/188.7)

Maclure Creek

Maclure Lake 11461'

11500

Mount Maclure 12910'

Mount Lyell 13114'

Ireland

11000

10500

Amelia Earhart Peak 11974'

Parsons Peak 12147'

Ireland Lake 10740'

1.5

Cathedral

11275'

Simmons Peak 12497'

12000

Range

Maclure Glacier

12500

11000

11500

11000

1 mile

1 kilometer

0.5

0.5

0

37.8°

37.78°

37.76°

37.74°

-119.2°

-119.22°

-119.24°

-119.26°

-119.28°

-119.3°

23

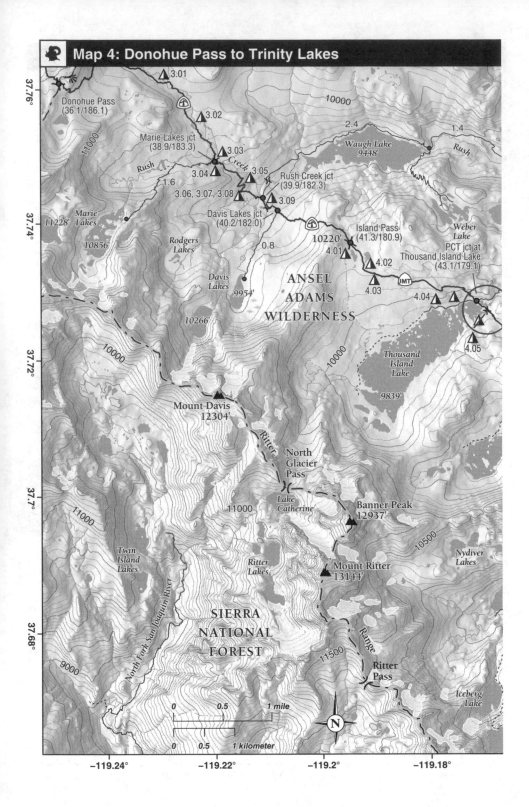

3.01

Donohue Pass
(36.1/186.1)

3.02

Marie Lakes jct
(38.9/183.3)

3.03

3.04   3.05

3.06, 3.07, 3.08

Rush Creek jct
(39.9/182.3)

3.09

Davis Lakes jct
(40.2/182.0)

Rush

Creek

1.6

10000

2.4

Waugh Lake
9448'

1.4

Rush

Weber
Lake

Island Pass
(41.3/180.9)

PCT jct at
Thousand Island Lake
(43.1/179.1)

10220'

4.01

4.02

4.03

JMT

4.04

ANSEL
ADAMS
WILDERNESS

0.8

Marie
11228'

Marie
Lakes

10856

Rodgers
Lakes

Davis
Lakes

9954'

10266'

Thousand
Island
Lake

9839'

4.05

10000

10000

Mount Davis
12304'

Ritter

North
Glacier
Pass

Lake
Catherine

11000

Banner Peak
12937'

10500

Nydiver
Lakes

Twin
Island
Lakes

Ritter
Lakes

Mount Ritter
13144'

SIERRA
NATIONAL
FOREST

11500

Range

Ritter
Pass

Iceberg
Lake

9000

North Fork San Joaquin River

11000

0   0.5   1 mile

N

0   0.5   1 kilometer

−119.24°   −119.22°   −119.2°   −119.18°

37.76°
37.74°
37.72°
37.7°
37.68°

24

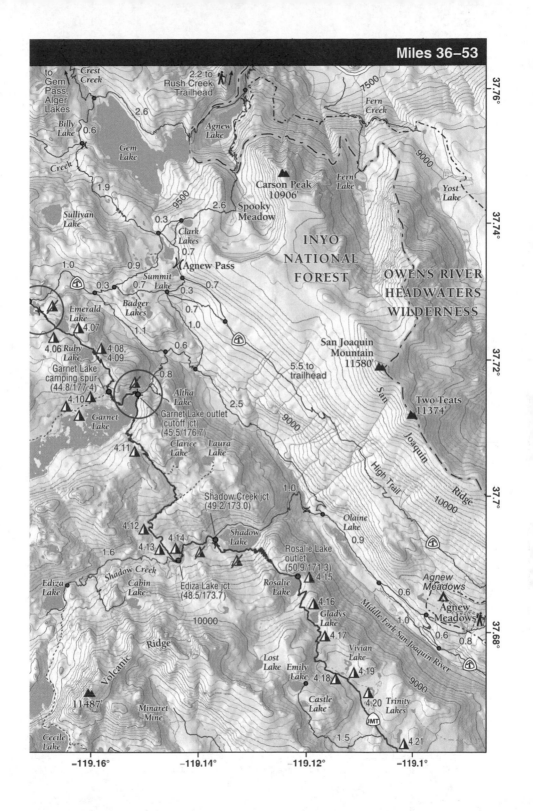

to Gem Pass, Alger Lakes

Crest Creek

2.2 to Rush Creek Trailhead

2.6

Billy Lake 0.6

Gem Lake

Agnew Lake

7500

Fern Creek

9000

Creek

1.9

Sullivan Lake

9500

2.6

Carson Peak 10906'

Spooky Meadow

Fern Lake

Yost Lake

0.3

Clark Lakes

1.0

0.9

Summit Lake

0.3

0.7

Agnew Pass

0.7

INYO NATIONAL FOREST

37.74°

0.3

Emerald Lake 4.07

Badger Lakes

0.7

0.7

OWENS RIVER HEADWATERS WILDERNESS

4.06 Ruby Lake

4.08, 4.09

1.1

1.0

San Joaquin Mountain 11580'

37.72°

Garnet Lake camping spur (44.8/177.4)

0.6

5.5 to trailhead

Two Teats 11374'

4.10

0.8

Altha Lake

Garnet Lake

Garnet Lake outlet (cutoff jct) (45.5/176.7)

2.5

9000

San

Joaquin

High Trail

Ridge

10000

4.11

Clarice Lake

Laura Lake

37.7°

1.0

Olaine Lake

Shadow Creek jct (49.2/173.0)

4.12

4.14

Shadow Lake

0.9

Agnew Meadows

4.13

1.6

Shadow Creek

Cabin Lake

Ediza Lake jct (48.5/173.7)

Rosalie Lake

Rosalie Lake outlet (50.9/171.3)

4.15

0.6

1.0

Middle Fork San Joaquin River

Agnew Meadows

Ediza Lake

0.6

0.8

10000

4.16

Gladys Lake

37.68°

Volcanic

Ridge

4.17

Vivian Lake

11487'

Minaret Mine

Lost Lake

Emily Lake

4.18

4.19

9000

Castle Lake

4.20

Trinity Lakes

Cecile Lake

JMT

1.5

4.21

-119.16° -119.14° -119.12° -119.1°

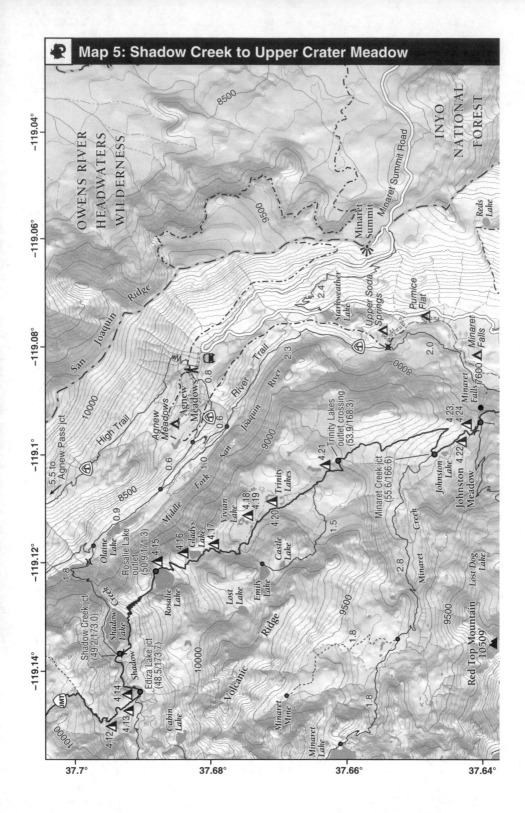

INYO NATIONAL FOREST

OWENS RIVER HEADWATERS WILDERNESS

Minaret Summit Road

8500

9500

9000

Reds Lake

Minaret Summit

Starkweather Lake

Upper Soda Springs

Pumice Flat

2.4

2.0

Minaret Falls

Minaret Falls 7600

San Joaquin Ridge

High Trail

River Trail

2.3

Agnew Pass jct

5.5 to

10000

0.8

Agnew Meadows

0.6

0.6

Agnew Meadows

Trinity Lakes outlet crossing (53.9/168.3)

Minaret Creek jct (55.6/166.6)

4.23, 4.24

1.0

San Joaquin River

4.21

Johnston Lake

Johnston 4.22 Meadow

8500

Middle Fork

9000

1.5

0.9

4.15

4.16

Gladys Lake

4.17

Vivian Lake

4.18 4.19

Trinity Lakes

4.20

Castle Lake

2.8

Minaret Creek

Lost Dog Lake

Olaine Lake

Rosalie Lake outlet (50.9/171.3)

Lost Lake

Emily Lake

Volcanic Ridge

9500

9500

1.8

Rosalie Lake

Red Top Mountain 10509

Shadow Creek jct (49.2/173.0)

1.8

Shadow Lake

10000

1.8

1.8

Shadow

Ediza Lake jct (48.5/173.7)

4.14

4.13

JMT

4.12

Cabin Lake

Minaret Mine

Minaret Lake

10000

37.7°   37.68°   37.66°   37.64°

-119.04°

-119.06°

-119.08°

-119.1°

-119.12°

-119.14°

26

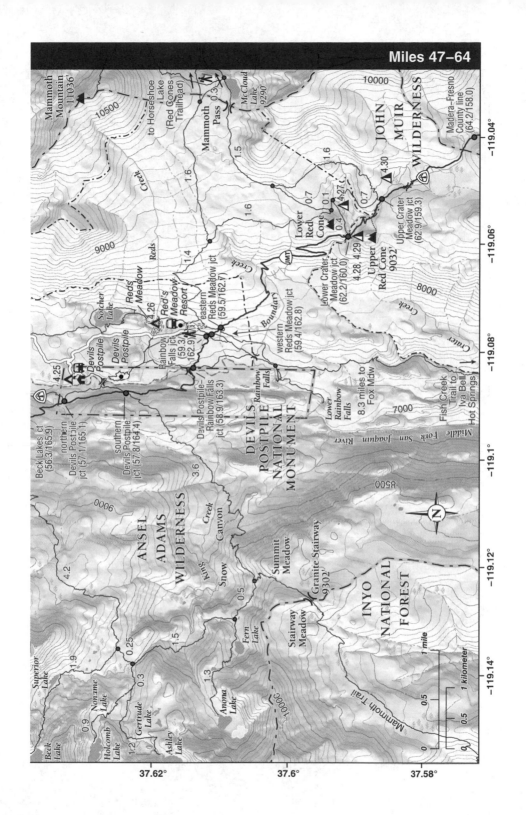

Mammoth Mountain 11036'

10500

to Horseshoe Lake (Red Cones Trailhead)

McCloud Lake 9290'

Mammoth Pass 0.3

Creek

1.5

1.6

10000

JOHN MUIR WILDERNESS

Madera–Fresno County line (64.2/158.0)

−119.04°

9000

1.6

1.6

1.6

▲4.30

−119.06°

Reds

1.4

Reds Meadow jct

Creek

0.7

0.1 ▲4.27

0.4

0.7

Lower Red Cone

Upper Crater Meadow jct (62.9/159.3)

−119.06°

Reds Meadow

4.26

Red's Meadow Resort

eastern Reds Meadow jct (59.5/162.7)

JMT

4.28, 4.29

Upper Red Cone 9032'

Lower Crater Meadow jct (62.2/160.0)

8000

Creek

Socher Lake

Devils Postpile

Rainbow Falls jct (59.3/162.9)

Boundary

western Reds Meadow jct (59.4/162.8)

−119.08°

4.25

Devils Postpile

Rainbow Falls

Lower Rainbow Falls

8.3 miles to Fox Mdw

Crater

Creek

Beck Lakes jct (56.3/165.9)

northern Devils Postpile jct (57.1/165.1)

southern Devils Postpile jct (57.8/164.4)

Devils Postpile–Rainbow Falls jct (58.9/163.3)

DEVILS POSTPILE NATIONAL MONUMENT

7000

Fish Creek Trail to Iva Bell Hot Springs

−119.1°

3.6

ANSEL

9000

4.2

ADAMS WILDERNESS

Kings

Creek

Canyon

Snow

Summit Meadow

Middle Fork San Joaquin River

8500

−119.12°

0.5

Granite Stairway 9302'

Stairway Meadow

INYO NATIONAL FOREST

N

Superior Lake

1.9

0.25

1.5

Fern Lake

1.3

Anona Lake

10000'

Mammoth Trail

1 mile

1 kilometer

0.5

0.5

−119.14°

Beck Lake

0.9

No-name Lake

Gertrude Lake

0.3

Holcomb Lake

1.2

Ashley Lake

37.62°

37.6°

37.58°

27

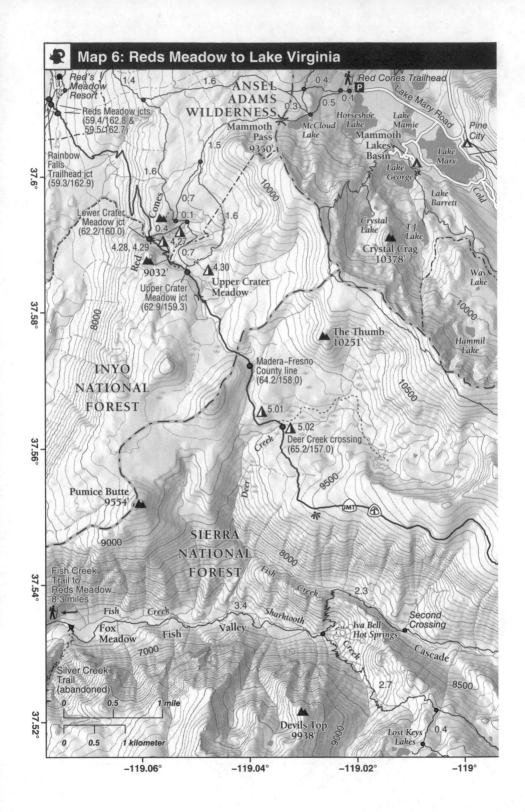

Red's Meadow Resort

1.4

1.6

ANSEL ADAMS WILDERNESS

0.4

Red Cones Trailhead

P

Lake Mary Road

Reds Meadow jcts (59.4/162.8 & 59.5/162.7)

0.3

0.5

0.1

McCloud Lake

Horseshoe Lake

Lake Mamie

Mammoth Lakes Basin

Pine City

Mammoth Pass 9350'

1.5

Lake George

Lake Mary

Rainbow Falls Trailhead jct (59.3/162.9)

1.6

1.6

10000

Lake Barrett

37.6°

Cones

0.7

Crystal Lake

T J Lake

Way Lake

Lower Crater Meadow jct (62.2/160.0)

0.1

0.4

1.6

Crystal Crag 10378'

4.28, 4.29

4.27

0.7

10000

Red

9032'

4.30

Upper Crater Meadow

Hammil Lake

Upper Crater Meadow jct (62.9/159.3)

37.58°

The Thumb 10251'

8000

INYO NATIONAL FOREST

Madera–Fresno County line (64.2/158.0)

10500

37.56°

5.01

5.02

Deer Creek crossing (65.2/157.0)

Deer Creek

9500

Pumice Butte 9554'

JMT

9000

SIERRA NATIONAL FOREST

Fish Creek

8000

Fish Creek Trail to Reds Meadow 8.3 miles

37.54°

2.3

Fish Creek

3.4

Sharktooth

Second Crossing

Fox Meadow

Valley

Fish

Iva Bell Hot Springs

Cascade

7000

Silver Creek Trail (abandoned)

8500

0   0.5   1 mile

2.7

37.52°

0   0.5   1 kilometer

Devils Top 9938'

9000

Lost Keys Lakes

0.4

−119.06°   −119.04°   −119.02°   −119°

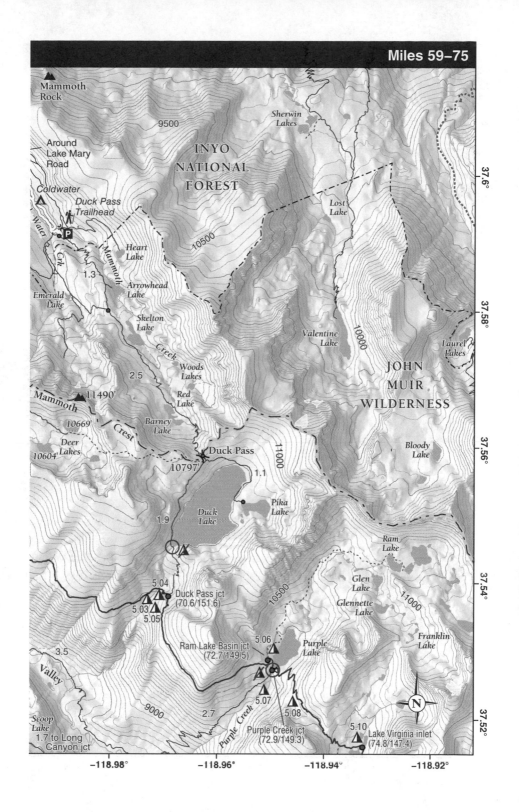

Mammoth Rock

Around Lake Mary Road

Coldwater

Duck Pass Trailhead

P

Water

Crk

Mammoth

1.3

Emerald Lake

Heart Lake

Arrowhead Lake

Skelton Lake

Creek

2.5

Woods Lakes

Red Lake

INYO NATIONAL FOREST

9500

10500

Sherwin Lakes

Lost Lake

Valentine Lake

10000

Laurel Lakes

JOHN MUIR WILDERNESS

Mammoth

10669'

11490'

Crest

Deer Lakes

10604'

Barney Lake

Duck Pass

10797

11000

1.1

Bloody Lake

Duck Lake

1.9

Píka Lake

Ram Lake

Glen Lake

Glennette Lake

11000

Franklin Lake

10500

5.04

Duck Pass jct (70.6/151.6)

5.03

5.05

3.5

Valley

9000

2.7

Scoop Lake

1.7 to Long Canyon jct

5.06

Ram Lake Basin jct (72.7/149.5)

5.07

Purple Creek

Purple Lake

5.08

Purple Creek jct (72.9/149.3)

5.10

Lake Virginia inlet (74.8/147.4)

N

37.6°

37.58°

37.56°

37.54°

37.52°

−118.98° −118.96° −118.94° −118.92°

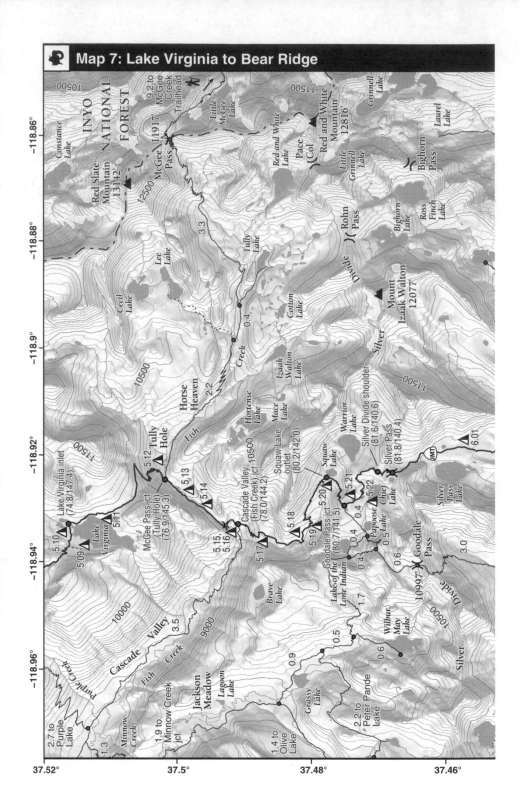

INYO NATIONAL FOREST

Constance Lake

10500

9.2 to McGee Creek Trailhead

Little McGee Lake

11500

Grinnell Lake

Laurel Lake

McGee 11917 Pass

Red and White Lake

Red and White Mountain 12816

Pace Col

Little Grinnell Lake

Bighorn Lake

Bighorn Pass

Red Slate Mountain 13142'

12500

Ross Finch Lake

Lee Lake

Tully Lake

Rohn Pass

Cecil Lake

3.3

Cotton Lake

Divide

Mount Izaak Walton 12077'

Creek

0.4

Izaak Walton Lake

Silver

10500

2.2

Horse Heaven

Hortense Lake

Mace Lake

Warrior Lake

11500

Silver Divide shoulder (81.6/140.6)

Fish

5.12 Tully Hole

Squaw Lake outlet (80.2/142.0)

Squaw Lake

Silver Pass (81.8/140.4)

Silver Pass Lake

6.01

11500

Lake Virginia inlet (74.8/147.4)

5.13

5.14

Cascade Valley (Fish Creek) jct 10500 (78.0/144.2)

5.18

5.20

5.21

5.22

Chief Lake

JMT

Silver Pass Lake

McGee Pass jct (Tully Hole) (76.9/145.3)

5.11

5.19

Goodale Pass jct (80.7/141.5)

Paapoose Lake

0.4

Lake Virginia

5.10

5.15, 5.16

0.4

0.5

5.09

5.17

Lake of the Lone Indian

0.4

Goodale Pass

3.0

Brave Lake

0.6

10997'

Divide

10000

9000

1.7

Wilbur May Lake

10500

Cascade Valley

3.5

Jackson Meadow

0.5

Grassy Lake

0.6

Silver

Purple Creek

Fish Creek

Lagoon Lake

0.9

2.7 to Purple Lake

1.3

Minnow Creek

1.9 to Minnow Creek jct

1.4 to Olive Lake

2.2 to Peter Pande Lake

—118.86°

—118.88°

—118.9°

—118.92°

—118.94°

—118.96°

37.52°

37.5°

37.48°

37.46°

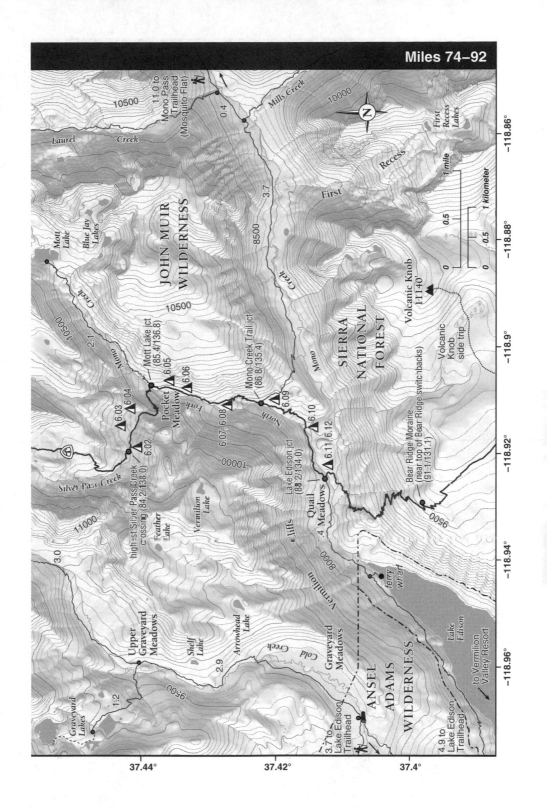

JOHN MUIR WILDERNESS

SIERRA NATIONAL FOREST

ANSEL ADAMS WILDERNESS

Mono Pass Trailhead (Mosquito Flat)
11.0 to

Laurel Creek

Mills Creek

10500

10000

First Recess Lakes

Recess

First

1 mile
1 kilometer
0.5
0.5
0

Mott Lake
Blue Jay Lakes

Mono Creek

8500

3.7

0.4

Volcanic Knob 11140'

Volcanic Knob side trip

Mott Lake jct (85.4/136.8)
6.05
6.06
2.1
Mono Creek

10500

Mono Creek Trail jct (86.8/135.4)
6.09

Bear Ridge Moraine (near top of Bear Ridge switchbacks) (91.1/131.1)

6.03
6.04

Fork

Pocket Meadow
6.07, 6.08
North
6.10
6.11, 6.12
9500

6.02
highest Silver Pass Creek crossing (84.2/138.0)
10000

Lake Edison jct (88.2/134.0)

Silver Pass Creek

3.0
Feather Lake
Vermilion Lake

Quail Meadows

11000

cliffs

Vermilion

8000

ferry wharf

Upper Graveyard Meadows

Shelf Lake
2.9
Arrowhead Lake

Cold Creek

Graveyard Meadows

Lake Edison

Graveyard Lakes
1.2

9500

3.7 to Lake Edison Trailhead

4.9 to Lake Edison Trailhead

to Vermilion Valley Resort

37.44°
37.42°
37.4°

–118.86°
–118.88°
–118.9°
–118.92°
–118.94°
–118.96°

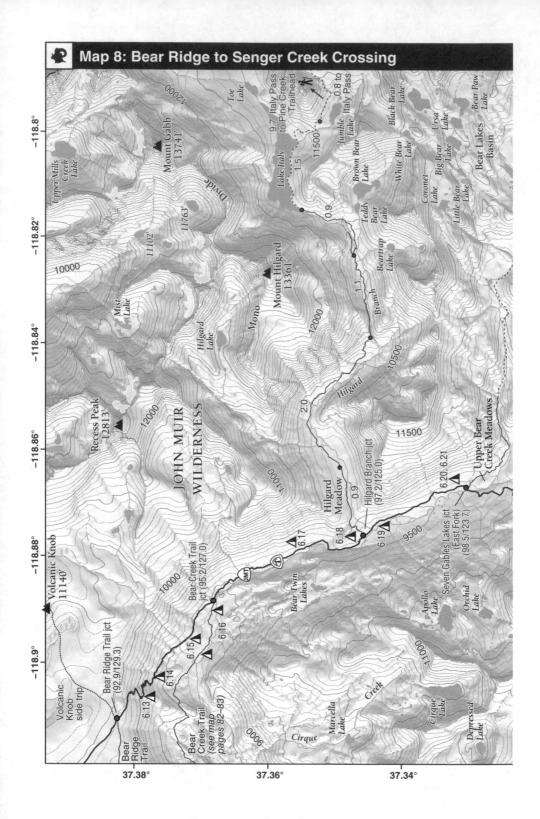

Toe
Lake

12000

9.7 Italy Pass
to Pine Creek
Trailhead

0.8 to
Italy Pass

N

Black Bear
Lake

Bear Paw
Lake

Mount Gabb
13741'

Jumble
Lake

Brown Bear
Lake

11500

Ursa
Lake

Bear Lakes
Basin

Lake Italy

White Bear
Lake

Big Bear
Lake

Upper Mills
Creek
Lake

Divide

1.5

Coronet
Lake

Little Bear
Lake

0.9

11763'

Teddy
Bear
Lake

11102

Bearrrap
Lake

10000

Mist
Lake

Mount Hilgard
13361'

1.1

Branch

Hilgard
Lake

Mono

12000

10500

Recess Peak
12813'

JOHN MUIR
WILDERNESS

Hilgard

2.0

11500

12000

11000

Hilgard
Meadow

Upper Bear
Creek Meadows

0.9

Hilgard Branch jct
(97.2/125.0)

6.20 6.21

6.18

6.17

9500

6.19

Volcanic Knob
11140'

10000

Bear Creek Trail
jct (95.2/127.0)

Seven Gables Lakes jct
(East Fork)
(98.5/123.7)

JMT

Bear Twin
Lakes

Apollo
Lake

Orchid
Lake

6.16

Bear Ridge Trail jct
(92.9/129.3)

6.15

11000

6.14

Creek

Cirque
Lake

Volcanic
Knob
side trip

6.13

Depressed
Lake

Bear
Ridge
Trail

Bear
Creek Trail
(see map
pages 82–83)

9000

Marcella
Lake

Cirque

9000

37.38°

37.36°

37.34°

–118.8°

–118.82°

–118.84°

–118.86°

–118.88°

–118.9°

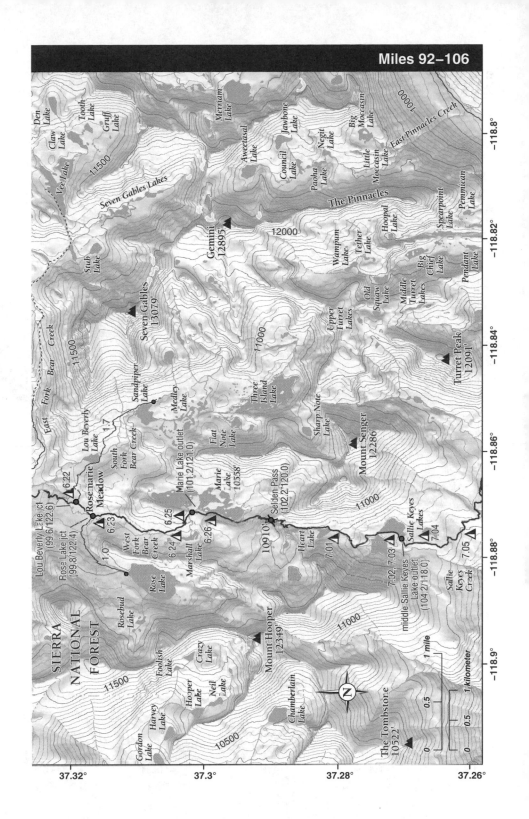

Den Lake

Tooth Lake

Claw Lake

Gruff Lake

Vee Lake

Merriam Lake

Jawbone Lake

Big Moccasin Lake

East Pinnacles Creek

10000

Aweetasal Lake

Council Lake

Negit Lake

Little Moccasin Lake

Spearpoint Lake

Pemmican Lake

Paoha Lake

Seven Gables Lakes

The Pinnacles

11500

Stub Lake

Hoopal Lake

Tether Lake

Wampum Lake

12000

Gemini 12895'

Big Chief Lake

Pendant Lake

Middle Turret Lakes

Old Squaw Lake

Upper Turret Lakes

Seven Gables 13079'

Sandpiper Lake

East Fork Bear Creek

11500

Medley Lake

11000

Turret Peak 12091'

Three Island Lake

South Fork Bear Creek

Lou Beverly Lake

1.7

Sharp Note Lake

Flat Note Lake

Marie Lake outlet (101.2/121.0)

Marie Lake 10558'

Mount Senger 12286'

6.22

Rosemarie Meadow

Selden Pass (102.2/120.0)

11000

Sallie Keyes Lakes

7.04

Lou Beverly Lake jct (99.6/122.6)

6.23

6.25

Heart Lake

7.01

Rose Lake jct (99.8/122.4)

6.24

6.26

10910'

7.05

West Fork Bear Creek

Marshall Lake

1.0

7.02, 7.03

middle Sallie Keyes Lake outlet (104.2/118.0)

Rose Lake

Rosebud Lake

SIERRA NATIONAL FOREST

11000

Sallie Keyes Creek

Foolish Lake

Crazy Lake

Mount Hooper 12349'

11500

Hooper Lake

Neil Lake

Chamberlain Lake

Harvey Lake

Gordon Lake

10500

11000

The Tombstore 10522'

1 mile

1 kilometer

0.5

0.5

1

0

0

-118.8°

-118.82°

-118.84°

-118.86°

-118.88°

-118.9°

37.32°

37.3°

37.28°

37.26°

33

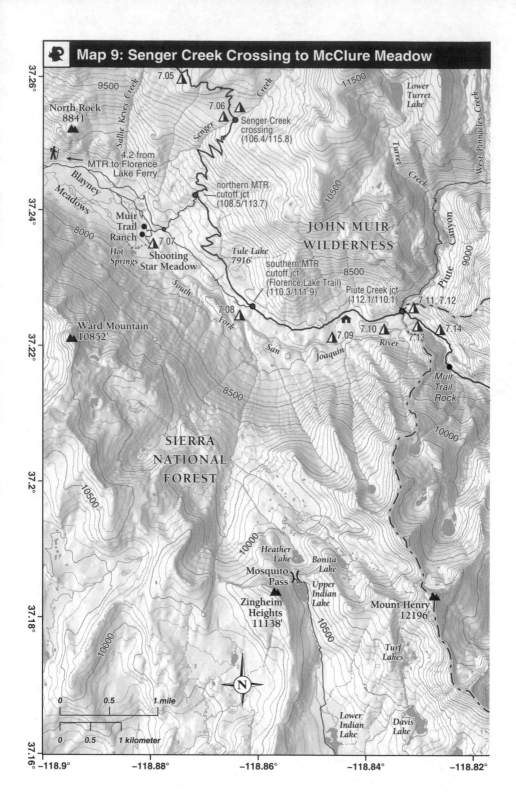

9500

7.05

Sallie Keyes Creek

Senger Creek

11500

Lower Turret Lake

North Rock 8841'

7.06

Senger Creek crossing (106.4/115.8)

West Pinnacles Creek

4.2 from MTR to Florence Lake Ferry

Senger

northern MTR cutoff jct (108.5/113.7)

Turret Creek

Blayney Meadows

10500

JOHN MUIR WILDERNESS

Piute Canyon

8000

Muir Trail Ranch

7.07

9000

Hot Springs

Shooting Star Meadow

Tule Lake 7916'

southern MTR cutoff jct (Florence Lake Trail) (110.3/111.9)

8500

Piute Creek jct (112.1/110.1)

7.11, 7.12

South Fork

7.08

7.14

Ward Mountain 10852'

San

7.09

7.10

River

7.13

Joaquin

Muir Trail Rock

8500

10000

SIERRA NATIONAL FOREST

10500

10000

10000

Heather Lake

Bonita Lake

Mosquito Pass

Upper Indian Lake

Zingheim Heights 11138'

Mount Henry 12196'

10500

Turf Lakes

N

0   0.5   1 mile

0   0.5   1 kilometer

Lower Indian Lake

Davis Lake

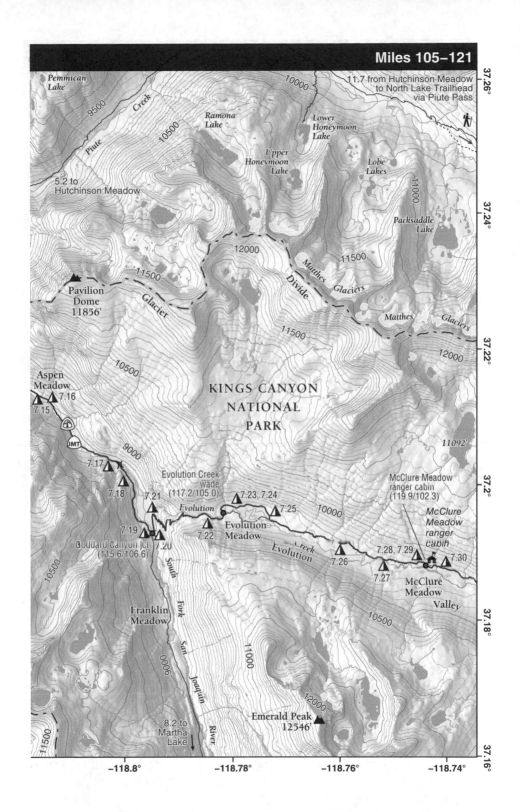

Pemmican Lake

Piute Creek

9500

10500

Ramona Lake

Lower Honeymoon Lake

Upper Honeymoon Lake

Lobe Lakes

11000

11.7 from Hutchinson Meadow to North Lake Trailhead via Piute Pass

Packsaddle Lake

37.26°

37.24°

5.2 to Hutchinson Meadow

Pavilion Dome 11856'

11500

Glacier

Matthes Glaciers

Divide

11500

12000

Matthes

Glaciers

11500

12000

37.22°

Aspen Meadow 7.16

7.15

JMT

10500

9000

7.17

7.18

7.21

7.19

Goddard Canyon Jct 7.20 (115.6/106.6)

KINGS CANYON NATIONAL PARK

Evolution Creek wade (117.2/105.0)

Evolution

7.22

Evolution Meadow

7.23, 7.24

7.25

10000

Evolution Creek

11092'

McClure Meadow ranger cabin (119.9/102.3)

McClure Meadow ranger cabin

7.28, 7.29

7.26

7.27

7.30

McClure Meadow Valley

37.2°

37.18°

Franklin Meadow

South Fork San Joaquin River

0006

10500

1000

11000

10500

12000

Emerald Peak 12546'

8.2 to Martha Lake

11500

37.16°

−118.8°   −118.78°   −118.76°   −118.74°

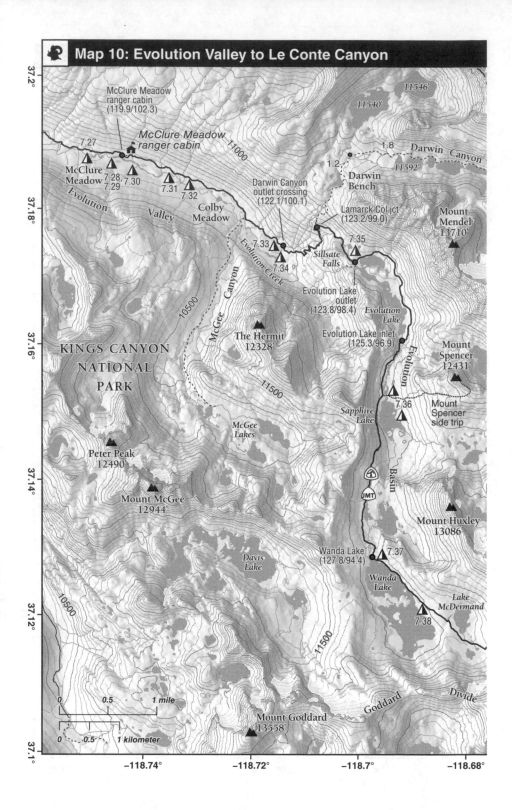

11546'

11540'

McClure Meadow
ranger cabin
(119.9/102.3)

7.27

*McClure Meadow
ranger cabin*

1.8

Darwin Canyon

1.2

11592'

Darwin
Bench

*McClure
Meadow*

7.28
7.29

7.30

Evolution

7.31

7.32

Darwin Canyon
outlet crossing
(122.1/100.1)

Lamarck Col jct
(123.2/99.0)

Mount
Mendel
13710'

*Colby
Meadow*

Valley

7.33

Evolution Creek

7.34

7.35

*Sillsate
Falls*

11000

McGee Canyon

10500

Evolution Lake
outlet
(123.8/98.4)

*Evolution
Lake*

KINGS CANYON
NATIONAL
PARK

The Hermit
12328'

Evolution Lake inlet
(125.3/96.9)

Mount
Spencer
12431'

11500

*Sapphire
Lake*

7.36

Mount
Spencer
side trip

Evolution

*McGee
Lakes*

Peter Peak
12490'

Basin

Mount McGee
12944'

JMT

Mount Huxley
13086'

*Davis
Lake*

Wanda Lake
(127.8/94.4)

7.37

10500

*Wanda
Lake*

*Lake
McDermand*

7.38

11500

Goddard

Divide

Mount Goddard
13558'

0   0.5   1 mile

0   0.5   1 kilometer

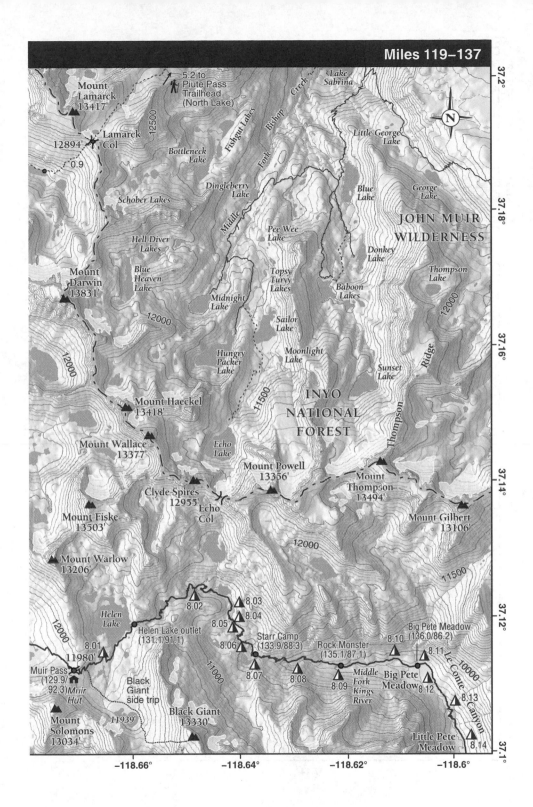

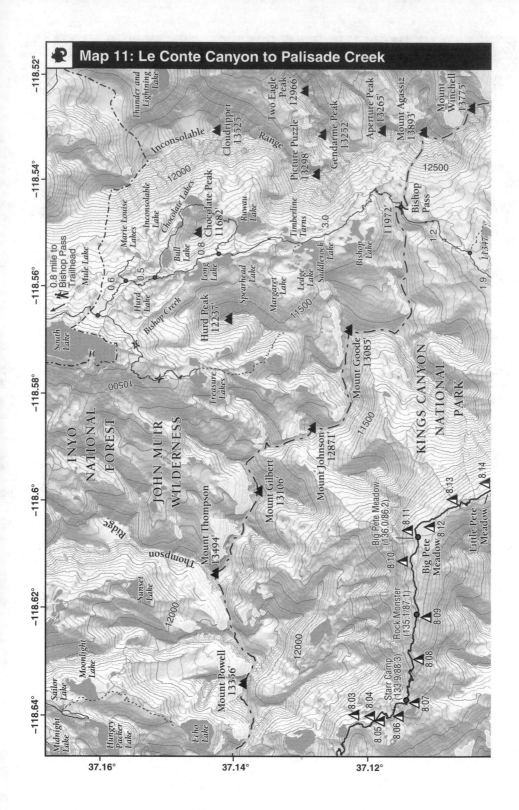

Thunder and Lightning Lake

Inconsolable Range

Cloudripper 13525'

Two Eagle Peak 12966'

Picture Puzzle 13298'

Gendarme Peak 13252

Aperture Peak 13265'

Mount Agassiz 13893'

Mount Winchell 1375'

12000

12500

Marie Louise Lakes

Inconsolable Lake

Chocolate Lakes

Chocolate Peak 11682

Ruwau Lake

Timberline Tarns

3.0

Bishop Pass

11972

Mule Lake

Bull Lake

Long Lake

Spearhead Lake

Margaret Lake

Ledge Lake

Saddlerock Lake

Bishop Lake

1.2

0.8 mile to Bishop Pass Trailhead

Hurd Lake

0.5

0.6

0.8

Bishop Creek

Hurd Peak 12237'

11500

11347'

1.9

South Lake

10500

Treasure Lakes

Mount Goode 13085

KINGS CANYON NATIONAL PARK

INYO NATIONAL FOREST

11500

JOHN MUIR WILDERNESS

Mount Johnson 12871

8.14

Mount Gilbert 13106'

8.13

Big Pete Meadow (136.0/86.2)

8.11

Thompson Ridge

Mount Thompson 13494

Little Pete Meadow

8.10

8.12

Big Pete Meadow

Sunset Lake

12000

Rock Monster (135.1/87.1)

8.09

8.08

Moonlight Lake

Mount Powell 13356'

12000

Starr Camp (133.9/88.3)

8.07

8.03

8.04

Sailor Lake

8.05

8.06

Midnight Lake

Hungry Packer Lake

Echo Lake

−118.52°
−118.54°
−118.56°
−118.58°
−118.6°
−118.62°
−118.64°

37.16°
37.14°
37.12°

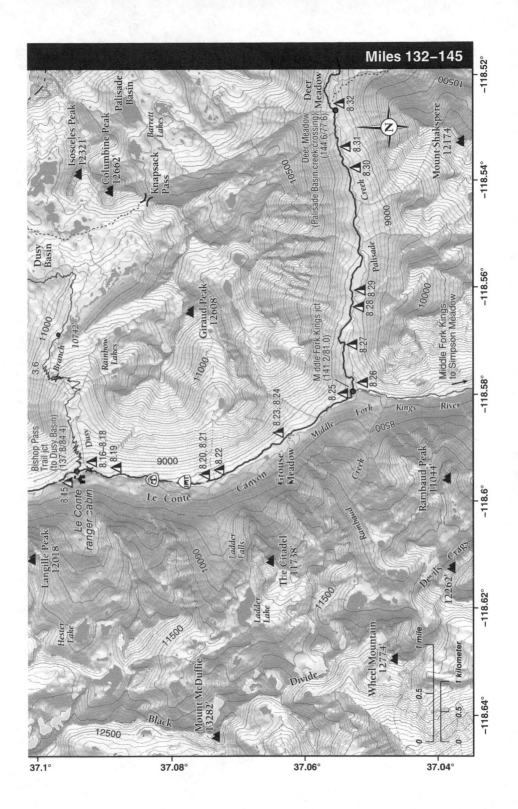

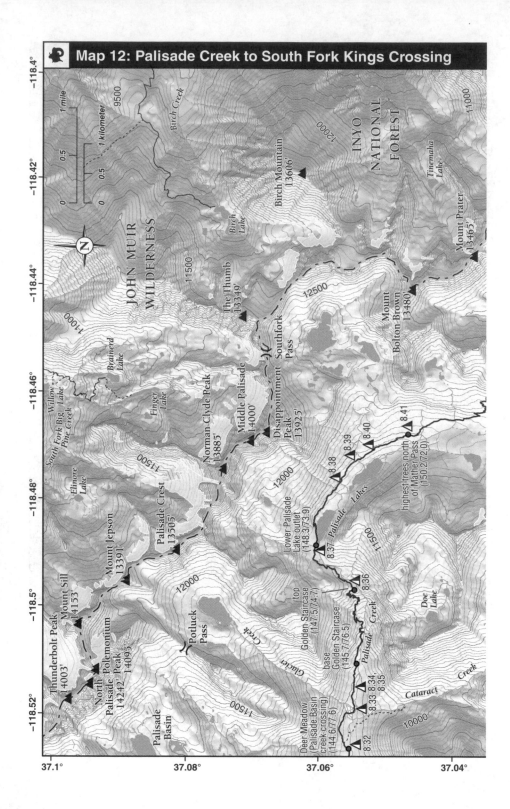

JOHN MUIR WILDERNESS

INYO NATIONAL FOREST

1 mile

1 kilometer

0.5

0.5

0

0

N

9500

Birch Creek

Birch Mountain
13606'

Birch Lake

Tinemaha Lake

Mount Prater
13465'

12000

11500

11000

The Thumb
13349'

12500

Southfork Pass

Mount Bolton-Brown
13480'

11000

Brainerd Lake

Finger Lake

Norman-Clyde Peak
13885'

Middle Palisade
14000'

Disappointment Peak
13925'

8.41

highest trees north
of Mather Pass
(150.2/72.0)

8.40

8.39

Willow Lake

South Fork Big Pine Creek

11500

8.38

Palisade Lakes

Elinore Lake

11500

12000

Lower Palisade
Lake outlet
(148.3/73.9)

8.31

Mount Jepson
13391'

Palisade Crest
13505'

8.37

Doe Lake

11500

Mount Sill
14153'

12000

top
Golden Staircase
(147.5/74.7)

8.36

Palisade Creek

Thunderbolt Peak
14003'

North Palisade
14242'

Polemonium Peak
14095'

Potluck Pass

Creek

Glacier Creek

base
Golden Staircase
(145.7/76.5)

Golden Staircase
(144.6/77.6)

8.33 8.34
8.35

Cataract Creek

10000

Palisade Basin

11500

Deer Meadow
(Palisade Basin
creek-crossing)

8.32

37.1°   37.08°   37.06°   37.04°

-118.4°
-118.42°
-118.44°
-118.46°
-118.48°
-118.5°
-118.52°

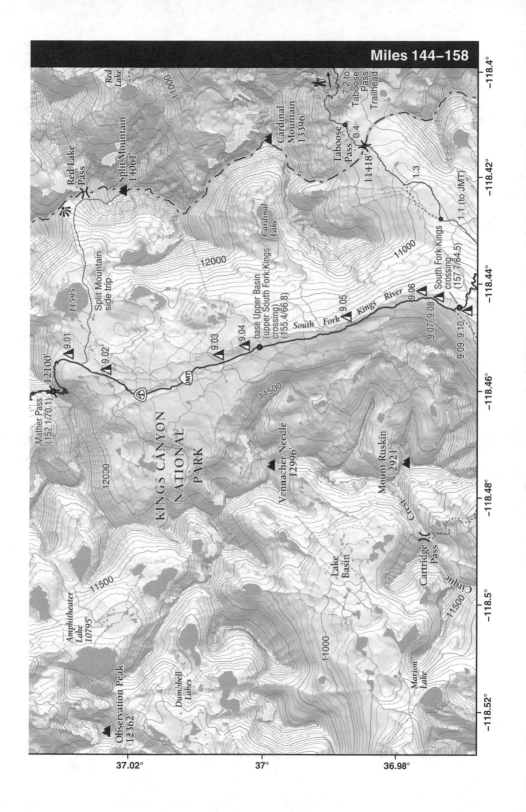

Red Lake

Split Mountain
14061'

Red Lake
Pass

Cardinal
Mountain
13396'

7.2 to
Taboose
Pass
Trailhead

Taboose
Pass

0.4

11418'

1.3

1.1 (to JMT)

Split Mountain
side trip

11595'

12000

Cardinal
Lake

Upper Basin
(upper South Fork Kings
crossing)
(155.4/66.8)

11000

South Fork Kings
crossing
(157.7/64.5)

9.01

9.02

9.03

9.04

base

9.05

South Fork Kings River

9.06

9.07, 9.08

9.09, 9.10,

12100'

Mather Pass
(152.1/70.1)

JMT

KINGS CANYON
NATIONAL
PARK

11500

Vennacher Needle
12996'

Mount Ruskin
2921'

12000

Crest

Cartridge Pass

11500

Amphitheater
Lake
10795'

11500

Lake
Basin

Cirque

Dumbbell
Lakes

11000

Marion
Lake

Observation Peak
12362'

37.02°

37°

36.98°

−118.4°

−118.42°

−118.44°

−118.46°

−118.48°

−118.5°

−118.52°

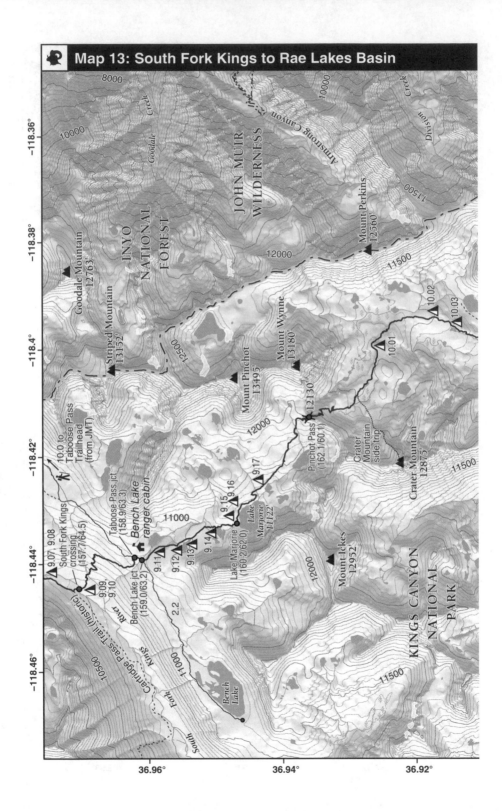

8000

Goodale Creek

10000

JOHN MUIR WILDERNESS

Armstrong Canyon

Division Creek

10000

INYO NATIONAL FOREST

Goodale Mountain 12763

Striped Mountain 13152'

11500

Mount Perkins 12560

12000

11500

10.02

10.03

Mount Wynne 13180'

10.01

Mount Pinchot 13495'

12130

10.0 to Taboose Pass Trailhead (from JMT)

12000

Pinchot Pass (162.1/60.1)

Crater Mountain side trip

Crater Mountain 12875

11500

Taboose Pass Jct (158.9/63.3)

Bench Lake ranger cabin

9.17

9.16

11000

9.15

Lake Marjorie 11122'

South Fork Kings crossing (157.7/64.5)

9.07, 9.08

9.14

Lake Marjorie (160.2/62.0)

Mount Ickes 12952

12000

KINGS CANYON NATIONAL PARK

9.11

9.12

9.13

Bench Lake Jct (159.0/63.2)

9.09, 9.10

2.2

11000

11500

Cartridge Pass Trail (historic)

10500

South Fork Kings River

Bench Lake

South

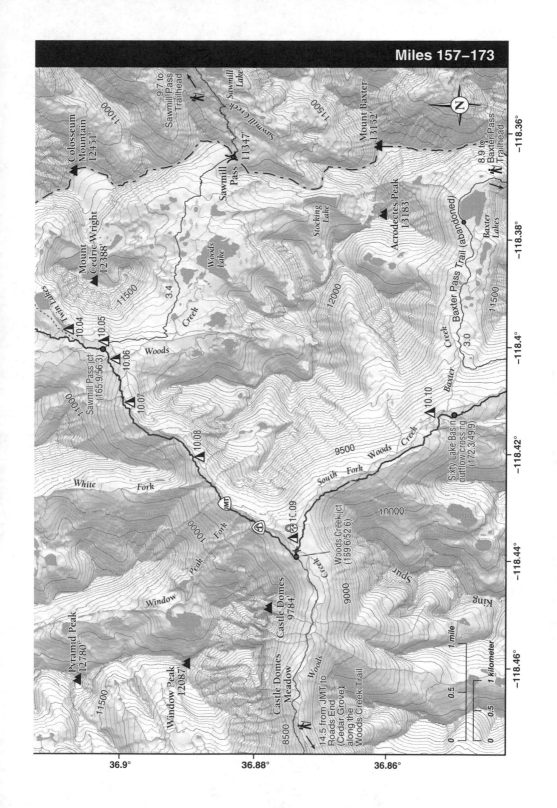

Colosseum
Mountain
12451'

11000

Sawmill Pass
Trailhead
9.7 to

Sawmill
Lake

Sawmill Creek

11500

Mount Baxter
13152'

8.9 to
Baxter Pass
Trailhead

Sawmill
Pass
11347'

Mount
Cedric Wright
12388'

Stocking
Lake

Acrodectes Peak
13183

Baxter Pass Trail (abandoned)

Baxter
Lakes

11500

11500

Woods
Lake

3.4

12000

3.0

Creek

Twin Lakes

10.04

10.05

10.06

Woods

Baxter

Creek

Sawmill Pass jct
(165.9/56.3)

10.07

11000

10.10

10.08

9500

Woods

Creek

Sixth Lake Basin
outflow crossing
(172.3/49.9)

White

Fork

South

Fork

10000

JMT

10.09

Woods Creek jct
(169.6/52.6)

Fork

10000

Pyramid Peak
12780'

Peak

Window

Castle Domes
9784'

9000

9000

Creek

King

Spur

Window Peak
12087'

11500

Castle Domes
Meadow

8500

Woods

14.5 from JMT to
Roads End
(Cedar Grove)
along the
Woods Creek Trail

1 mile

1 kilometer

0.5

0.5

0

0

36.9°

36.88°

36.86°

−118.36°

−118.38°

−118.4°

−118.42°

−118.44°

−118.46°

43

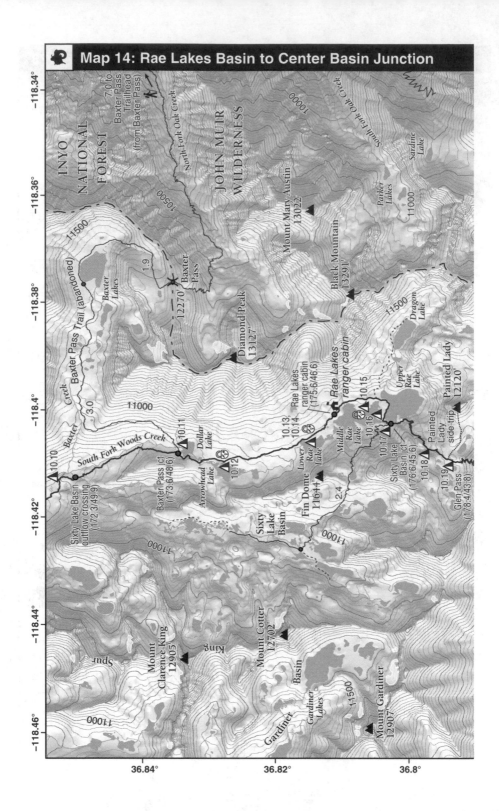

INYO NATIONAL FOREST

JOHN MUIR WILDERNESS

7.0 to Baxter Pass Trailhead (from Baxter Pass)

North Fork Oak Creek

South Fork Oak Creek

Sardine Lake

10000

Parker Lakes

11000

Mount Mary Austin 13022'

Black Mountain 13291'

Baxter Pass Trail (abandoned)

11500

1.9

Baxter Lakes

Baxter Pass

12270'

Diamond Peak 13127'

Dragon Lake

11500

Rae Lakes

Upper Rae Lake

Painted Lady 12120'

Creek

3.0

11000

Baxter Creek

South Fork Woods Creek

Dollar Lake

10.11

Rae Lakes ranger cabin

10.13

10.14

Rae Lakes ranger cabin (175.6/46.6)

10.15

10.16

10.17

Painted Lady side-trip

10.18

Arrowhead Lake

10.12

Lower Rae Lake

Middle Rae Lake

Sixty Lake Basin jct (176.6/45.6)

10.10

Baxter Pass jct (173.6/48.6)

Sixty Lake Basin outflow crossing (172.3/49.9)

Fin Dome 11644'

2.4

Glen Pass (178.4/43.8)

10.19

Sixty Lake Basin

11000

11000

King

Spur

Mount Clarence King 12905'

Mount Cotter 12702'

Gardiner Basin

Gardiner Lakes

11500

Mount Gardiner 12907'

11000

10000

36.84°
36.82°
36.8°

-118.34°
-118.36°
-118.38°
-118.4°
-118.42°
-118.44°
-118.46°

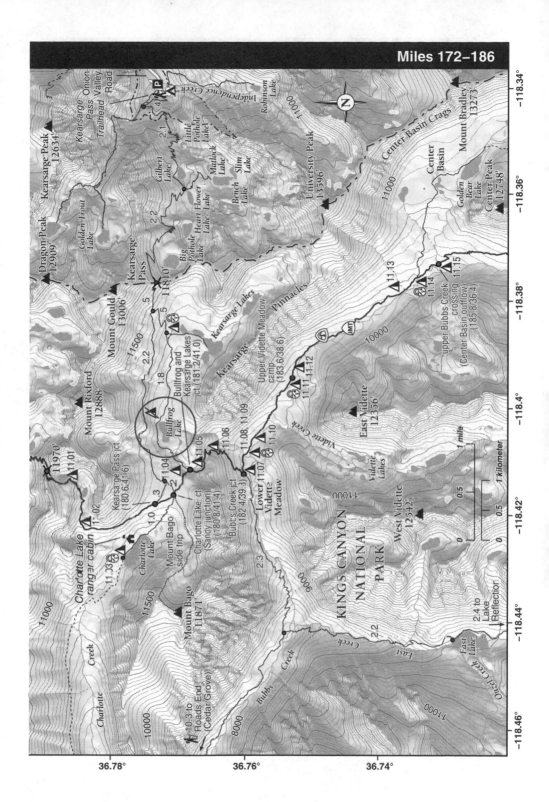

Kearsarge Onion Valley
Pass- Road
Trailhead

Independence Creek

P
.4

2.1

Robinson Lake

Mount Bradley 13273

Center Basin Crags

Kearsarge Peak 12634

Kearsarge Pass- Trailhead

Gilbert Lake

Little Pothole Lake

Matlock Lake

Bench Lake

Slim Lake

University Peak 13596

Center Basin

Mount Bradley 13273

Dragon Peak 12909

Golden Trout Lake

2.2

Heart Lake

Flower Lake

Golden Bear Lake

Center Peak 12748

Kearsarge Pass

Mount Gould 13006

.5

11810'

Big Pothole Lake

Kearsarge Lakes

Pinnacles

11.13

upper Bubbs Creek crossing (185.8/36.4)

11.15

11.14

5

Bullfrog and Kearsarge Lakes jct (181.2/41.0)

Kearsarge

Upper Vidette Meadow camp (183.6/38.6)

10000

Center Basin outflow (185.8/36.4)

11500

2.2

1.8

Mount Rixford 12888'

Bullfrog Lake

11.06

11.08 11.09

11.10

JMT

11.11 11.12

East Vidette 12356'

Vidette Creek

1 mile

1197 0'

11.01

Kearsarge Pass jct (180.6/41.6)

11.04

11.05

Bubbs Creek jct (182.4/39.3)

Lower Vidette Meadow

1.07

1 kilometer

11000

Vidette Lakes

1.02

.2

.3

1.0

Charlotte Lake jct (Sandy junction) (180.8/41.4)

2.3

West Vidette 12542'

0.5

0.5

Charlotte Lake ranger cabin

11.38

Charlotte Lake

Mount Bago side trip

KINGS CANYON NATIONAL PARK

0

0

1-500

9006

2.4 to Lake Reflection

Charlotte Creek

Mount Bago 11871'

East Creek

2.2

East Lake

Onon Creek

10.3 to Roads End (Cedar Grove)

8000

Bubbs Creek

11000

10000

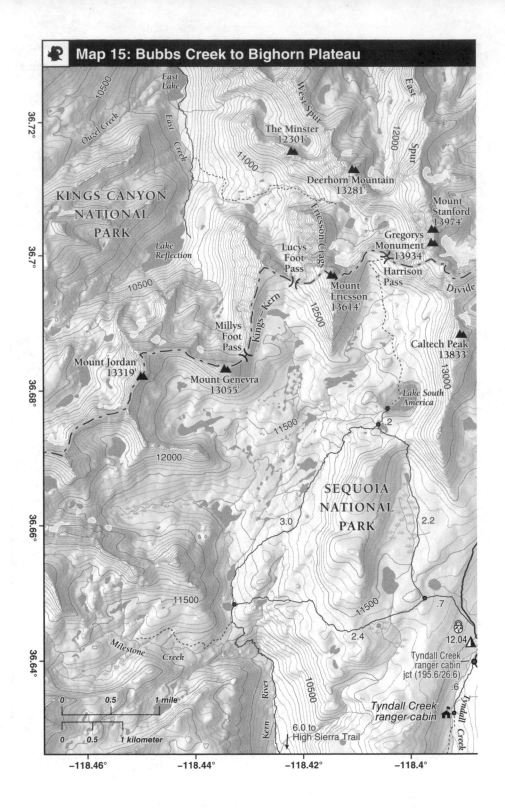

KINGS CANYON
NATIONAL
PARK

SEQUOIA
NATIONAL
PARK

East Lake

West Spur

East Spur

Ouzel Creek

East Creek

Lake Reflection

The Minster
12301'

Deerhorn Mountain
13281'

Mount Stanford
13974'

Gregorys Monument
13934'

Harrison Pass

Ericsson Crags

Lucys Foot Pass

Mount Ericsson
13614'

Divide

Caltech Peak
13833'

Millys Foot Pass

Kings–Kern

Mount Jordan
13319'

Mount Genevra
13055'

Lake South America

.2

3.0

2.2

2.2

.7

12.04

Tyndall Creek ranger cabin jct (195.6/26.6)

.6

Tyndall Creek ranger cabin

Milestone Creek

Kern River

Tyndall Creek

6.0 to High Sierra Trail

10500

12000

11000

10500

10500

12500

11500

12000

11500

11500

11500

13000

10500

0   0.5   1 mile

0   0.5   1 kilometer

36.72°
36.7°
36.68°
36.66°
36.64°

−118.46°   −118.44°   −118.42°   −118.4°

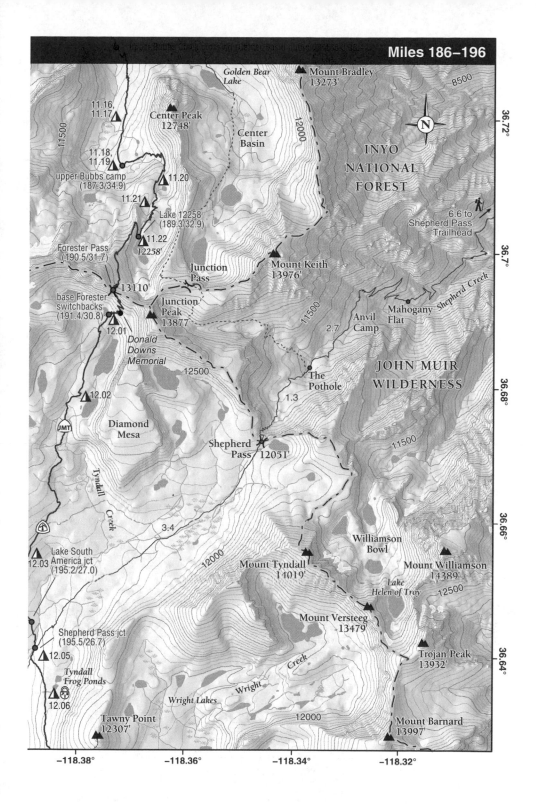

Mount Bradley
13273'

Golden Bear
Lake

8500

12000

INYO
NATIONAL
FOREST

11500

11.16,
11.17

Center Peak
12748'

Center
Basin

N

6.6 to
Shepherd Pass
Trailhead

36.72°

11.18,
11.19

11.20

upper Bubbs camp
(187.3/34.9)

11.21

Lake 12258
(189.3/32.9)

11.22

12258'

Mount Keith
13976'

Junction
Pass

36.7°

Forester Pass
(190.5/31.7)

13110'

Junction
Peak
13877

Shepherd Creek

base Forester
switchbacks
(191.4/30.8)

12.01

Donald
Downs
Memorial

11500

Mahogany
Flat

Anvil
Camp

2.7

JOHN MUIR
WILDERNESS

36.68°

12.02

12500

The
Pothole

1.3

11500

JMT

Diamond
Mesa

Shepherd Pass 12051'

Tyndall Creek

3.4

36.66°

12.03

Lake South
America jct
(195.2/27.0)

12000

Williamson
Bowl

Mount Tyndall
14019'

Lake
Helen of Troy

Mount Williamson
14389'

12500

Shepherd Pass jct
(195.5/26.7)

12.05

Mount Versteeg
13479'

Trojan Peak
13932'

36.64°

Tyndall
Frog Ponds

12.06

Wright Creek

Tawny Point
12307'

Wright Lakes

12000

Mount Barnard
13997'

−118.38° −118.36° −118.34° −118.32°

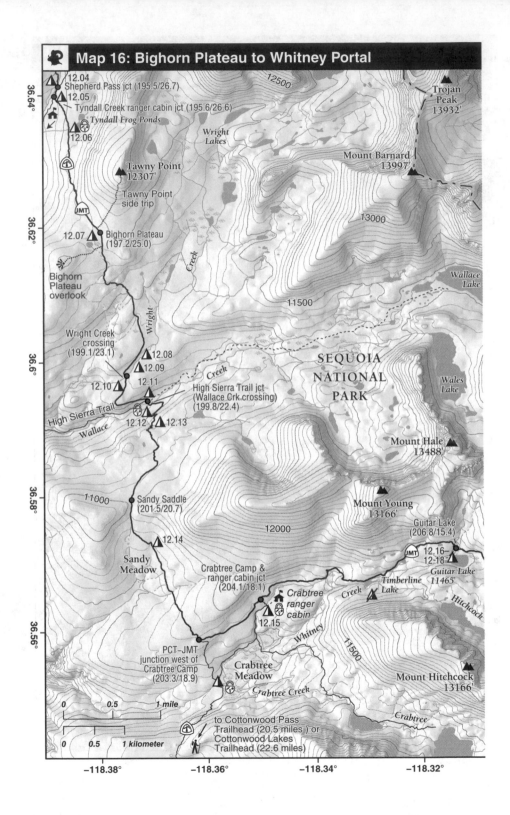

Map 16: Bighorn Plateau to Whitney Portal

12.04
Shepherd Pass jct (195.5/26.7)

12.05
Tyndall Creek ranger cabin jct (195.6/26.6)

Tyndall Frog Ponds

12.06

12500

Trojan Peak 13932'

Wright Lakes

Tawny Point 12307'

Mount Barnard 13997'

Tawny Point side trip

JMT

13000

12.07 Bighorn Plateau (197.2/25.0)

Creek

Wallace Lake

Bighorn Plateau overlook

11500

Wright Creek crossing (199.1/23.1)

Wright

12.08
12.09
12.11

SEQUOIA NATIONAL PARK

Wales Lake

12.10

Creek

High Sierra Trail jct (Wallace Crk.crossing) (199.8/22.4)

High Sierra Trail

Wallace

12.12   12.13

Mount Hale 13488'

11000

Sandy Saddle (201.5/20.7)

Mount Young 13166'

Guitar Lake (206.8/15.4)

12000

12.14

JMT   12.16–
12.18

Sandy Meadow

Crabtree Camp & ranger cabin jct (204.1/18.1)

Timberline Lake

Creek

Guitar Lake 11465'

Hitchcock

Crabtree ranger cabin

12.15

Whitney

11500

PCT–JMT junction west of Crabtree Camp (203.3/18.9)

Crabtree Meadow

Mount Hitchcock 13166'

Crabtree Creek

0   0.5   1 mile

Crabtree

0   0.5   1 kilometer

to Cottonwood Pass Trailhead (20.5 miles) or Cottonwood Lakes Trailhead (22.6 miles)

36.64°
36.62°
36.6°
36.58°
36.56°

−118.38°   −118.36°   −118.34°   −118.32°

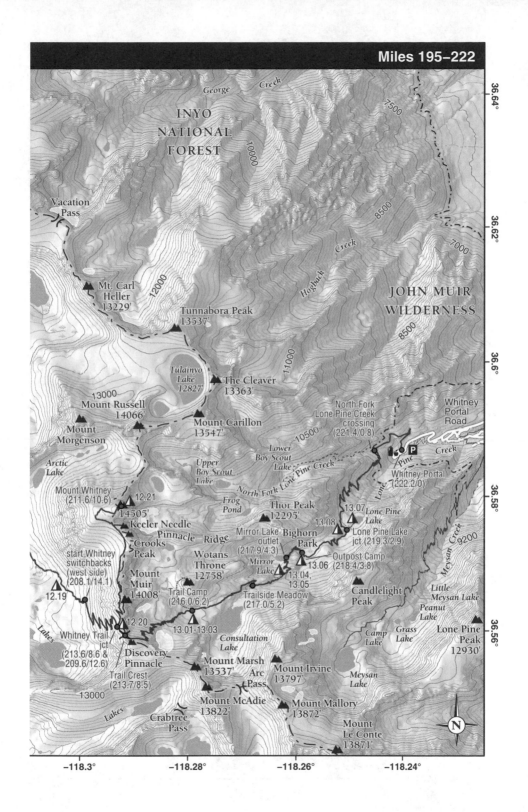

George Creek

INYO
NATIONAL
FOREST

7500

10000

Vacation
Pass

8500

7000

Hogback Creek

Mt. Carl
Heller
13229'

12000

Tunnabora Peak
13537'

JOHN MUIR
WILDERNESS

8500

Tulainyo
Lake
12827'

The Cleaver
13363'

11000

13000

Mount Russell
14066'

Mount Carillon
13547'

10500

North Fork
Lone Pine Creek
crossing
(221.4/0.8)

Whitney
Portal
Road

Mount
Morgenson

Arctic
Lake

Upper
Boy Scout
Lake

Lower
Boy Scout
Lake

North Fork Lone Pine Creek

Pine Creek

Whitney Portal
(222.2/0)

Mount Whitney
(211.6/10.6)

12.21

14505'

Keeler Needle

Pinnacle Ridge

Crooks
Peak

Frog
Pond

Thor Peak
12295'

Mirror Lake
outlet
(217.9/4.3)

Bighorn
Park

13.07

13.08

Lone Pine
Lake

Lone Pine Lake
jct (219.3/2.9)

Meysan Creek

9200

start Whitney
switchbacks
(west side)
(208.1/14.1)

12.19

Mount
Muir
14008'

Wotans
Throne
12758'

Mirror
Lake

13.04
13.05

13.06

Outpost Camp
(218.4/3.8)

Candlelight
Peak

Little
Meysan
Lake

Peanut
Lake

Trail Camp
(216.0/6.2)

Trailside Meadow
(217.0/5.2)

Lakes

12.20

Whitney Trail
jct
(213.6/8.6 &
209.6/12.6)

Discovery
Pinnacle

13.01-13.03

Consultation
Lake

Camp
Lake

Grass
Lake

Lone Pine
Peak
12930'

Trail Crest
(213.7/8.5)

13000

Mount Marsh
13537'

Arc
Pass

Mount Irvine
13797'

Meysan
Lake

Lakes

Crabtree
Pass

Mount McAdie
13822'

Mount Mallory
13872'

Mount
Le Conte
13871'

N

−118.3° −118.28° −118.26° −118.24°

36.64°
36.62°
36.6°
36.58°
36.56°

Happy Isles to Tuolumne–Mariposa County Line:
MERCED RIVER (18.1 miles)

Location	Elevation	Distance from Previous Point	Cumulative Distance	Latitude, Longitude
Happy Isles mileage sign	4,060'	–	0	37.73052°N, 119.55801°W
Vernal Fall bridge	4,420'	0.7	0.7	37.72612°N, 119.55168°W
base Mist Trail junction	4,540'	0.2	0.9	37.72625°N, 119.54851°W
Clark Point junction	5,490'	1.0	1.9	37.72503°N, 119.54498°W
Panorama Trail junction	5,980'	1.0	2.9	37.72259°N, 119.53484°W
top Mist Trail junction	5,980'	0.4	3.3	37.72623°N, 119.53042°W
Half Dome–Merced Lake junction (west end LYV)	6,120'	0.6	3.9	37.73072°N, 119.52296°W
northeastern corner Little Yosemite Valley (junction)	6,130'	0.6	4.5	37.73452°N, 119.51502°W
Half Dome junction	6,990'	1.4	5.9	37.74507°N, 119.51276°W
Clouds Rest junction	7,180'	0.5	6.4	37.74410°N, 119.50374°W
Merced High Trail junction	7,950'	2.0	8.4	37.75634°N, 119.47900°W
Forsyth Trail junction	8,010'	0.1	8.5	37.75740°N, 119.47867°W
highest Sunrise Creek crossing	8,540'	1.7	10.2	37.76532°N, 119.45301°W
Sunrise Lakes junction (Sunrise High Sierra Camp)	9,320'	2.8	13.0	37.79347°N, 119.43315°W
Echo Creek junction	9,330'	0.9	13.9	37.80306°N, 119.43018°W
Cathedral Pass	9,710'	2.6	16.5	37.83481°N, 119.41538°W
Lower Cathedral Lake junction	9,440'	1.1	17.6	37.84824°N, 119.41478°W
Merced–Tuolumne drainage divide	9,570'	0.5	18.1	37.85380°N, 119.41299°W

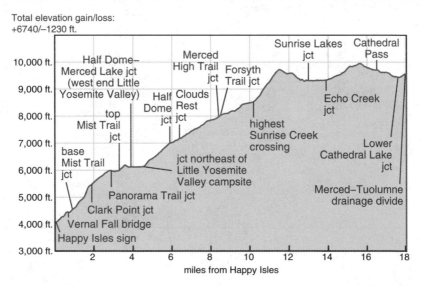

Total elevation gain/loss:
+6740/−1230 ft.

miles from Happy Isles

Tuolumne–Mariposa County Line to Donohue Pass:
TUOLUMNE RIVER (18.0 miles)

Location	Elevation	Distance from Previous Point	Cumulative Distance	Latitude, Longitude
Merced–Tuolumne drainage divide	9,570'	–	18.1	37.85380°N, 119.41299°W
Cathedral Lakes Trailhead junction (western Tuolumne Meadows perimeter trail junction)	8,600'	2.4	20.5	37.87202°N, 119.38386°W
leave Tuolumne Meadows perimeter trail	8,640'	0.8	21.3	37.87026°N, 119.37166°W
Parsons Lodge junction	8,570'	0.6	21.9	37.87787°N, 119.36611°W
CA 120 crossing at Lembert Dome	8,600'	0.8	22.7	37.87704°N, 119.35308°W
Dog Lake parking area junction (Lembert Dome side trip)	8,660'	0.9	23.6	37.87717°N, 119.33839°W
Tuolumne Lodge junction	8,700'	0.1	23.7	37.87598°N, 119.33540°W
Gaylor Lakes junction	8,710'	0.1	23.8	37.87568°N, 119.33412°W
eastern merge with Tuolumne Meadows perimeter trail	8,660'	0.6	24.4	37.86876°N, 119.33358°W
Rafferty Creek junction	8,710'	0.7	25.1	37.86677°N, 119.32307°W
Evelyn & Ireland Lakes junction	8,910'	4.3	29.4	37.82554°N, 119.27966°W
Lyell Forks	9,010'	3.0	32.4	37.78973°N, 119.26205°W
upper Lyell Fork bridge	9,650'	1.1	33.5	37.77765°N, 119.26211°W
upper Lyell camp	10,190'	0.9	34.4	37.76796°N, 119.25656°W
Donohue Pass	11,060'	1.7	36.1	37.76101°N, 119.24872°W

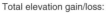

Total elevation gain/loss:
+3090/−1620 ft.

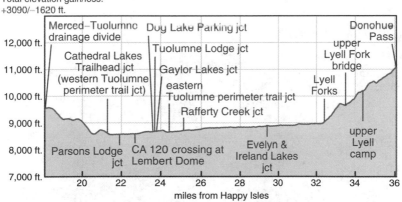

Section 3
Donohue Pass to Island Pass:
RUSH CREEK (5.2 miles)

Location	Elevation	Distance from Previous Point	Cumulative Distance	Latitude, Longitude
Donohue Pass	11,060'	–	36.1	37.76101°N, 119.24872°W
Marie Lakes junction	10,060'	2.8	38.9	37.74934°N, 119.22032°W
Rush Creek junction	9,640'	1.0	39.9	37.74389°N, 119.21127°W
Davis Lakes junction	9,700'	0.3	40.2	37.74198°N, 119.20849°W
Island Pass	10,220'	1.1	41.3	37.73705°N, 119.19471°W

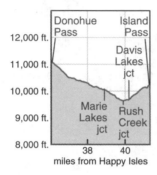

Donohue Pass
Island Pass
Davis Lakes jct
Marie Lakes jct
Rush Creek jct

12,000 ft.
11,000 ft.
10,000 ft.
9,000 ft.
8,000 ft.

38   40
miles from Happy Isles

Total elevation gain/loss:
+2090/–3570 ft.

Panorama south from Donohue Pass

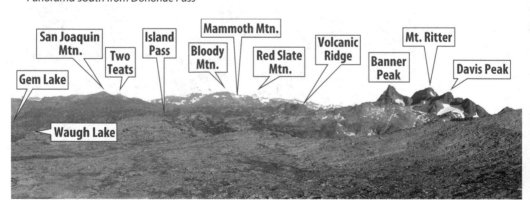

San Joaquin Mtn.
Two Teats
Island Pass
Mammoth Mtn.
Bloody Mtn.
Red Slate Mtn.
Volcanic Ridge
Mt. Ritter
Banner Peak
Davis Peak
Gem Lake
Waugh Lake

Section 4

Island Pass to Madera–Fresno County Line:
MIDDLE FORK OF THE SAN JOAQUIN RIVER

(22.9 miles)

Location	Elevation	Distance from Previous Point	Cumulative Distance	Latitude, Longitude
Island Pass	10,220'	–	41.3	37.73705°N, 119.19471°W
PCT junction at Thousand Island Lake	9,850'	1.8	43.1	37.72851°N, 119.17130°W
Garnet Lake camping spur	9,940'	1.7	44.8	37.71529°N, 119.15660°W
Garnet Lake outlet (River Trail cutoff junction)	9,680'	0.7	45.5	37.71487°N, 119.15123°W
Ediza Lake junction	9,010'	3.0	48.5	37.69043°N, 119.14367°W
Shadow Creek junction at Shadow Lake	8,770'	0.7	49.2	37.69349°N, 119.13667°W
Rosalie Lake outlet	9,340'	1.7	50.9	37.68810°N, 119.12148°W
Trinity Lakes outlet crossing	9,000'	3.0	53.9	37.66133°N, 119.10097°W
Minaret Creek junction (Johnston Meadow)	8,130'	1.7	55.6	37.64708°N, 119.09979°W
Beck Lakes junction	8,100'	0.7	56.3	37.64034°N, 119.09382°W
northern Devils Postpile junction	7,680'	0.8	57.1	37.63292°N, 119.08901°W
southern Devils Postpile junction	7,720'	0.7	57.8	37.62377°N, 119.08752°W
Devils Postpile–Rainbow Falls junction	7,480'	1.1	58.9	37.61393°N, 119.08283°W
Rainbow Falls Trailhead junction	7,630'	0.4	59.3	37.61201°N, 119.07698°W
western Reds Meadow junction	7,650'	0.1	59.4	37.61120°N, 119.07662°W
eastern Reds Meadow junction	7,720'	0.1	59.5	37.60988°N, 119.07536°W
Lower Crater Meadow junction	8,650'	2.7	62.2	37.59115°N, 119.05852°W
Upper Crater Meadow junction	8,920'	0.7	62.9	37.58623°N, 119.05150°W
Madera–Fresno County Line	9,220'	1.3	64.2	37.57250°N, 119.03987°W

Total elevation gain/loss:
+4320/–5330 ft.

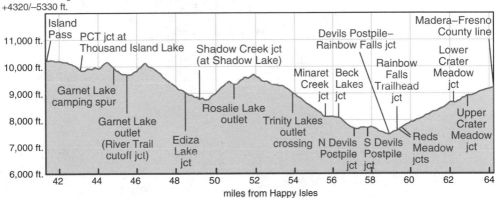

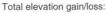

Section 5

Madera–Fresno County Line to Silver Pass:
FISH CREEK BRANCH OF THE MIDDLE FORK
OF THE SAN JOAQUIN RIVER (17.6 miles)

Location	Elevation	Distance from Previous Point	Cumulative Distance	Latitude, Longitude
Madera–Fresno County Line	9,220'	–	64.2	37.57250°N, 119.03987°W
Deer Creek crossing	9,110'	1.0	65.2	37.56355°N, 119.03375°W
Duck Pass junction	10,170'	5.4	70.6	37.53833°N, 118.96913°W
Ram Lake Basin junction (Purple Lake west shore)	9,980'	2.1	72.7	37.52898°N, 118.95031°W
Purple Creek junction (to Cascade Valley)	9,940'	0.2	72.9	37.52750°N, 118.94950°W
Lake Virginia inlet	10,350'	1.9	74.8	37.51621°N, 118.93286°W
McGee Pass junction (Tully Hole)	9,530'	2.1	76.9	37.50168°N, 118.92461°W
Cascade Valley (Fish Creek) junction	9,200'	1.1	78.0	37.49111°N, 118.93289°W
Squaw Lake* outlet	10,290'	2.2	80.2	37.47780°N, 118.92426°W
Goodale Pass junction	10,540'	0.5	80.7	37.47505°N, 118.92946°W
Silver Divide shoulder	10,940'	0.9	81.6	37.46996°N, 118.92312°W
Silver Pass	10,740'	0.2	81.8	37.46770°N, 118.92315°W

*This lake's problematic name will likely change in the near future.

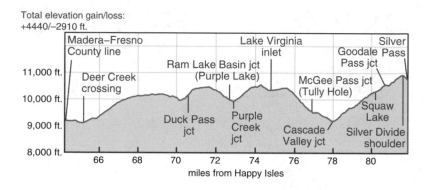

Total elevation gain/loss:
+4440/–2910 ft.

Section 6
Silver Pass to Selden Pass:
MONO AND BEAR CREEKS (20.4 miles)

Location	Elevation	Distance from Previous Point	Cumulative Distance	Latitude, Longitude
Silver Pass	10,740'	–	81.8	37.46770°N, 118.92315°W
highest Silver Pass Creek crossing	9,690'	2.4	84.2	37.44179°N, 118.91955°W
Mott Lake junction	9,020'	1.2	85.4	37.43851°N, 118.90730°W
Mono Creek Trail junction	8,350'	1.4	86.8	37.42221°N, 118.91052°W
Lake Edison (Quail Meadows) junction (to VVR & ferry)	7,900'	1.4	88.2	37.41259°N, 118.92470°W
Bear Ridge moraine (near top of Bear Ridge switchbacks)	9,560'	2.9	91.1	37.39795°N, 118.92968°W
Bear Ridge Trail junction	9,880'	1.8	92.9	37.38256°N, 118.91050°W
Bear Creek Trail junction	8,950'	2.3	95.2	37.36820°N, 118.88851°W
Hilgard Branch junction (to Italy Pass)	9,330'	2.0	97.2	37.34565°N, 118.87620°W
Seven Gables Lakes junction (East Fork Bear Creek)	9,580'	1.3	98.5	37.33030°N, 118.86717°W
Lou Beverly Lake junction	10,030'	1.1	99.6	37.31914°N, 118.86947°W
Rose Lake junction	10,040'	0.2	99.8	37.31665°N, 118.87215°W
Marie Lake outlet	10,550'	1.4	101.2	37.30166°N, 118.87148°W
Selden Pass	10,910'	1.0	102.2	37.28992°N, 118.87296°W

Total elevation gain/loss:
+4430/–4270 ft.

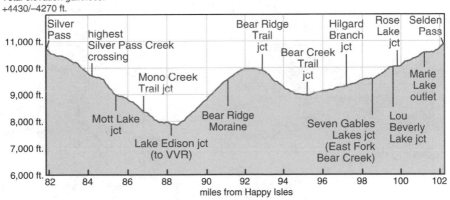

Selden Pass to Muir Pass:
SOUTH FORK OF THE SAN JOAQUIN RIVER
(27.7 miles)

Location	Elevation	Distance from Previous Point	Cumulative Distance	Latitude, Longitude
Selden Pass	10,910'	–	102.2	37.28992°N, 118.87296°W
middle Sallie Keyes Lake outlet	10,200'	2.0	104.2	37.27012°N, 118.87655°W
Senger Creek crossing	9,750'	2.2	106.4	37.25354°N, 118.86444°W
northern Muir Trail Ranch cutoff junction	8,410'	2.1	108.5	37.24221°N, 118.87184°W
southern MTR cutoff junction (Florence Lake Trail)	7,890'	1.8	110.3	37.22577°N, 118.86123°W
Piute Creek junction	8,080'	1.8	112.1	37.22511°N, 118.83350°W
Goddard Canyon junction	8,490'	3.5	115.6	37.19281°N, 118.79504°W
Evolution Creek wade	9,200'	1.6	117.2	37.19573°N, 118.78181°W
McClure Meadow ranger cabin	9,630'	2.7	119.9	37.18806°N, 118.74384°W
Darwin Canyon outflow crossing	9,950'	2.2	122.1	37.17455°N, 118.71392°W
Lamarck Col junction	10,640'	1.1	123.2	37.17730°N, 118.70757°W
Evolution Lake outlet	10,880'	0.6	123.8	37.17212°N, 118.70052°W
Evolution Lake inlet	10,870'	1.5	125.3	37.16058°N, 118.69187°W
Wanda Lake near outlet	11,430'	2.5	127.8	37.12863°N, 118.69732°W
Muir Pass	11,980'	2.1	129.9	37.11205°N, 118.67093°W

Total elevation gain/loss:
+5150/–4090 ft.

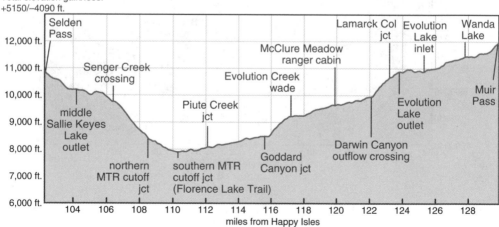

Muir Pass to Mather Pass:
MIDDLE FORK OF THE KINGS RIVER
(22.2 miles)

Location	Elevation	Distance from Previous Point	Cumulative Distance	Latitude, Longitude
Muir Pass	11,980'	–	129.9	37.11205°N, 118.67093°W
Helen Lake outlet	11,630'	1.2	131.1	37.11882°N, 118.65969°W
Starr Camp	10,330'	2.8	133.9	37.11434°N, 118.63712°W
Rock Monster	9,490'	1.2	135.1	37.11264°N, 118.62135°W
Big Pete Meadow (at creek crossing)	9,250'	0.9	136.0	37.11260°N, 118.60683°W
Bishop Pass Trail junction (to Dusy Basin)	8,750'	1.8	137.8	37.09414°N, 118.59433°W
Middle Fork Kings junction (to Simpson Meadow)	8,040'	3.4	141.2	37.05284°N, 118.57937°W
Deer Meadow (Palisade Basin creek crossing)	8,830'	3.4	144.6	37.05541°N, 118.52673°W
base Golden Staircase	9,060'	1.1	145.7	37.05423°N, 118.51094°W
top Golden Staircase	10,310'	1.8	147.5	37.05455°N, 118.49727°W
Lower Palisade Lake outlet	10,610'	0.8	148.3	37.06022°N, 118.48894°W
highest trees north of Mather Pass	10,980'	1.9	150.2	37.04660°N, 118.46817°W
Mather Pass	12,100'	1.9	152.1	37.03115°N, 118.46017°W

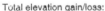

Total elevation gain/loss:
+4750/–4630 ft.

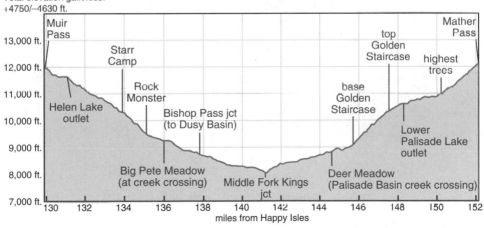

Section 9

Mather Pass to Pinchot Pass:
SOUTH FORK OF THE KINGS RIVER
(10.0 miles)

Location	Elevation	Distance from Previous Point	Cumulative Distance	Latitude, Longitude
Mather Pass	12,100'	–	152.1	37.03115°N, 118.46017°W
base Upper Basin (South Fork Kings crossing)	10,830'	3.3	155.4	37.00087°N, 118.45191°W
main South Fork Kings crossing	10,040'	2.3	157.7	36.97038°N, 118.44456°W
Taboose Pass junction	10,780'	1.2	158.9	36.96217°N, 118.43874°W
Bench Lake junction	10,770'	0.1	159.0	36.96110°N, 118.43921°W
Lake Marjorie	11,130'	1.2	160.2	36.94688°N, 118.43241°W
Pinchot Pass	12,130'	1.9	162.1	36.93604°N, 118.41257°W

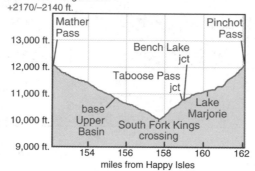

Total elevation gain/loss:
+2170/–2140 ft.

Panorama north from Mather Pass

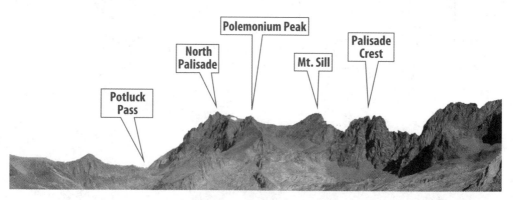

Pinchot Pass to Glen Pass:
WOODS CREEK BRANCH OF THE KINGS RIVER
(16.3 miles)

Location	Elevation	Distance from Previous Point	Cumulative Distance	Latitude, Longitude
Pinchot Pass	12,130'	–	162.1	36.93604°N, 118.41257°W
Sawmill Pass junction	10,370'	3.8	165.9	36.90262°N, 118.40041°W
Woods Creek junction	8,540'	3.7	169.6	36.87374°N, 118.43924°W
Sixty Lake Basin outflow crossing	9,520'	2.7	172.3	36.84991°N, 118.41260°W
Baxter Pass junction (Dollar Lake)	10,220'	1.3	173.6	36.83463°N, 118.40815°W
Rae Lakes ranger cabin	10,600'	2.0	175.6	36.81129°N, 118.40081°W
Sixty Lake Basin junction	10,560'	1.0	176.6	36.80274°N, 118.40255°W
Glen Pass	11,970'	1.8	178.4	36.78956°N, 118.41179°W

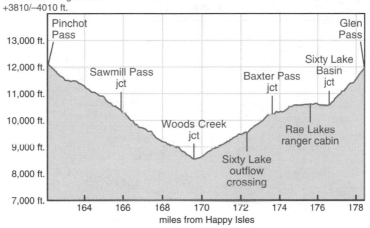

Total elevation gain/loss:
+3810/–4010 ft.

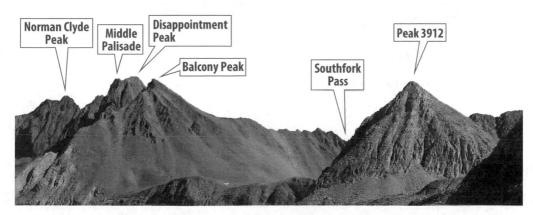

Section 11

Glen Pass to Forester Pass:
BUBBS CREEK BRANCH OF THE KINGS RIVER
(12.1 miles)

Location	Elevation	Distance from Previous Point	Cumulative Distance	Latitude, Longitude
Glen Pass	11,970'	–	178.4	36.78956°N, 118.41179°W
Kearsarge Pass junction	10,770'	2.2	180.6	36.77339°N, 118.41791°W
Charlotte Lake junction (Sandy Junction)	10,740'	0.2	180.8	36.77063°N, 118.41626°W
Bullfrog and Kearsarge Lakes junction	10,530'	0.4	181.2	36.76816°N, 118.41148°W
Bubbs Creek junction	9,560'	1.2	182.4	36.76024°N, 118.41229°W
Upper Vidette Meadow camp	9,910'	1.2	183.6	36.75295°N, 118.39428°W
upper Bubbs Creek crossing (Center Basin outflow)	10,530'	2.2	185.8	36.73093°N, 118.37311°W
upper Bubbs camp	11,230'	1.5	187.3	36.71308°N, 118.37188°W
Lake 12,258' (north of Forester Pass)	12,250'	2.0	189.3	36.70244°N, 118.36881°W
Forester Pass	13,110'	1.2	190.5	36.69452°N, 118.37351°W

Total elevation gain/loss:
+3700/–2530 ft.

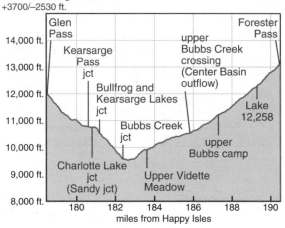

Forester Pass to Trail Crest:
KERN RIVER
(23.2 miles)

Location	Elevation	Distance from Previous Point	Cumulative Distance	Latitude, Longitude
Forester Pass	13,110'	–	190.5	36.69452°N, 118.37351°W
base Forester Pass switchbacks	12,500'	0.9	191.4	36.69088°N, 118.37430°W
Lake South America junction	11,040'	3.8	195.2	36.64516°N, 118.38816°W
Shepherd Pass junction	10,910'	0.3	195.5	36.64132°N, 118.38751°W
Tyndall Creek ranger cabin junction	10,880'	0.1	195.6	36.63985°N, 118.38824°W
Bighorn Plateau	11,440'	1.6	197.2	36.61927°N, 118.37994°W
Wright Creek crossing	10,700'	1.9	199.1	36.59805°N, 118.37510°W
High Sierra Trail junction (Wallace Creek crossing)	10,410'	0.7	199.8	36.59430°N, 118.37117°W
Sandy Saddle	10,980'	1.7	201.5	36.57960°N, 118.37431°W
PCT junction west of Crabtree camping area	10,770'	1.8	203.3	36.55890°N, 118.36180°W
Crabtree Camp (and ranger cabin)	10,700'	0.8	204.1	36.56479°N, 118.35040°W
Guitar Lake (Arctic Lake outlet creek crossing)	11,490'	2.7	206.8	36.57227°N, 118.31398°W
start Mount Whitney switchbacks	12,320'	1.3	208.1	36.56462°N, 118.29903°W
Mount Whitney Trail junction	13,460'	1.5	209.6	36.56060°N, 118.29303°W
Mount Whitney	14,505'	2.0	211.6	36.57852°N, 118.29227°W
Mount Whitney Trail junction	13,460'	2.0	213.6	36.56060°N, 118.29303°W
Trail Crest	13,610'	0.1	213.7	36.55933°N, 118.29156°W

Total elevation gain/loss:
+5850/–5380 ft.

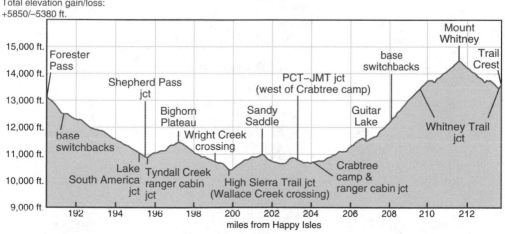

Trail Crest to Whitney Portal:
OWENS RIVER (8.5 miles)

Location	Elevation	Distance from Previous Point	Cumulative Distance	Latitude, Longitude
Trail Crest	13,610'	–	213.7	36.55933°N, 118.29156°W
Trail Camp	12,020'	2.3	216.0	36.56298°N, 118.27914°W
Trailside Meadow	11,360'	1.0	217.0	36.56670°N, 118.26800°W
Mirror Lake outlet	10,660'	0.9	217.9	36.57087°N, 118.26176°W
Outpost Camp	10,370'	0.5	218.4	36.57159°N, 118.25886°W
Lone Pine Lake junction	10,030'	0.9	219.3	36.57500°N, 118.25051°W
North Fork Lone Pine Creek crossing	8,730'	2.1	221.4	36.58682°N, 118.24539°W
Whitney Portal	8,330'	0.8	222.2	36.58692°N, 118.24019°W

Total elevation gain/loss:
+120/–5390 ft.

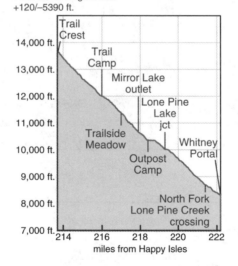

OPPOSITE: *Massive slab walls rise above Mirror Lake.*

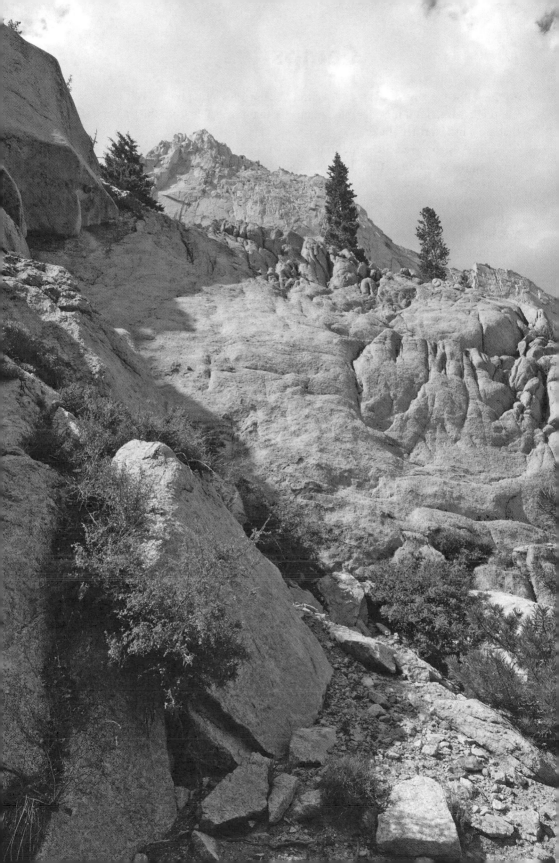

Campsites

The following table provides a selection of campsites along the JMT. It is not comprehensive, but it includes most campsites that are visible from the trail and some that are a little farther afield.

Campsites above treeline tend to be smaller and more hidden; a few are included here, but the selection of these high-elevation sites is more sparing to discourage large groups of people from converging on a location that is suitable for only a few tents. More choices are available with a little searching.

Remember: The coordinates indicate where you leave the trail, *not* where you camp. You must be 100 feet from trail and water to camp (or 25 feet for established campsites in Sequoia and Kings Canyon National Parks). If a campsite is located significantly off the trail and it might be unclear what location is being suggested, the actual campsite location is given in parentheses. Note that your GPS may also be off a little, so the onus is on you to use common sense and abide by LNT principles, so if you don't see somewhere sensible to camp, look a bit farther up or down the track.

Campsites where fires are not allowed are marked with an icon (🚫). North-to-south distances are in miles from Happy Isles, and south-to-north distances are in miles from Whitney Portal. These waypoints are also available for download at tinyurl.com /JMTWaypoints.

Camp ID	N–S	S–N	Elevation	Latitude, Longitude	Description
1.01	4.4	217.8	6,120'	37.73283°N, 119.51502°W	large camping area in eastern Little Yosemite Valley; toilet; food-storage boxes; currently unavailable for holders of Happy Isles to Donohue Pass permits
1.02	6.3	215.9	7,110'	37.74372°N, 119.50590°W	many small sites to the south of the trail in white fir–Jeffrey pine forest; good views to Half Dome
1.03	6.4	215.8	7,170'	37.74399°N, 119.50421°W	many small sites to the south of the trail in white fir–Jeffrey pine forest; also small sites on the knob to the northwest of the Clouds Rest junction
1.04	6.5	215.7	7,180'	37.74372°N, 119.50295°W	large camping area by Sunrise Creek; head south from the JMT along a use trail
1.05	6.6	215.6	7,260'	37.74441°N, 119.50175°W	site for several tents on knob with open Jeffrey pine cover and excellent views to Half Dome; head west from trail
1.06	6.9	215.3	7,390'	37.74410°N, 119.49666°W	sites for 3 tents on flat rib north and northwest of the trail, under surviving open Jeffrey pine–white fir cover
1.07	7.1	215.1	7,480'	37.74578°N, 119.49421°W	3 tent sites on open, sandy rib north of the trail with scattered surviving Jeffrey pines; vistas west; this site survives, but areas nearby are mostly burned (37.74602°N, 119.49475°W)
1.08	7.9	214.3	7,830'	37.75120°N, 119.48252°W	2 small tent sites in burned terrain east of trail; water to west in Sunrise Creek
1.09	9.6	212.6	8,430'	37.76119°N, 119.45925°W	3+ tent sites in flat, sandy openings to the north of the trail, toward Sunrise Creek; among red fir, western white pine, and lodgepole pine

Camp ID	N–S	S–N	Elevation	Latitude, Longitude	Description
1.10	10.1	212.1	8,500'	37.76319°N, 119.45310°W	large opening in red fir forest beside a Sunrise Creek tributary; may need to detour west to Sunrise Creek for water in late season
1.11	10.2	212.0	8,560'	37.76552°N, 119.45302°W	site for 6 tent sites in opening in red fir forest alongside Sunrise Creek; head west of the trail; additional sites farther upstream to the east of the trail
1.12 🐻	11.6	210.6	9,720'	37.77802°N, 119.44388°W	large, flat, sandy site among bedrock outcrops, big western white pine, and lodgepole pine; southeast of the trail; beautiful views; no water
1.13 🐻	11.8	210.4	9,600'	37.78055°N, 119.44139°W	site for 3–4 tents beneath open lodgepole pines at the edge of a large meadow; south of the trail; unreliable late-season water
1.14 🐻	12.0	210.2	9,570'	37.78135°N, 119.43821°W	site for 3–4 tents beneath open lodgepole pines at the edge of a large meadow; south of the trail; unreliable late-season water
1.15 🐻	12.1	210.1	9,590'	37.78257°N, 119.43624°W	large, flat, sandy site to the southeast of the trail under lodgepole pine and western white pine; beautiful views; no water
1.16	12.6	209.6	9,330'	37.78896°N, 119.43538°W	2–3 tent sites on a slight shelf, beneath hemlock and lodgepole pine; northeast of the trail and creek; excellent views to Mount Florence
1.17	13.0	209.2	9,320'	37.79346°N, 119.43315°W	Sunrise High Sierra Camp backpackers' camping area; large area with many tent sites, a water tap (very occasionally dry), and toilet; head a short distance along the trail toward Sunrise Lakes to reach the camping area (37.79405°N, 119.43411°W)
1.18	14.7	207.5	9,560'	37.81345°N, 119.42728°W	space for 3–4 tents in sandy sites on bedrock rib southeast of trail; small tarn nearby (37.81302°N, 119.42717°W)
1.19 🐻	15.7	206.5	9,950'	37.82348°N, 119.41726°W	space for many tents on a sandy shelf east of the trail with scattered lodgepole pine; view to Matthes Crest, Mount Clark, Mount Florence; no water
1.20 🐻	16.6	205.6	9,710'	37.83553°N, 119.41491°W	Cathedral Pass; sandy flats among lodgepole pines to the east of the trail; water usually available in meadows to the south; view to Mount Florence, Echo Peaks, Matthes Crest
1.21 🐻	17.1	205.1	9,610'	37.84112°N, 119.41323°W	northeast shore Upper Cathedral Lake; head southwest along a use trail to a few sandy sites among slab and in open lodgepole pine forest; ensure you are 100' from water, and do not camp in the meadow
1.22 🐻	17.6	204.6	9,300'	37.84820°N, 119.41474°W	north shore Lower Cathedral Lake; many picturesque sites in sandy patches in open forest; head 0.5 mile down the side trail (37.84615°N, 119.42546°W)
2.01	22.7	199.5	8,590'	37.87710°N, 119.35313°W	Tuolumne Meadows backpackers' campground; food-storage boxes, water, and toilets; $5 per person; actual backpacker' campsite location will have changed when campground reopens in 2024, following renovations (expected new location: 37.87710°N, 119.35313°W)
2.02	28.9	193.3	8,850'	37.83204°N, 119.28180°W	large area under open lodgepole pine cover west of the trail
2.03	29.3	192.9	8,870'	37.82713°N, 119.27966°W	space for 4+ tents in a little pocket of lodgepole pines above the trail; nice spot and next to a very scenic bit of river where the water flows over bedrock
2.04	29.4	192.8	8,900'	37.82554°N, 119.27966°W	large openings ringed by lodgepole pine forest to the northwest and southeast of the Evelyn Lake junction; campsite is in a slightly different location vs. previous editions of this book—the trail was moved and now passes through parts of the old site

Camp ID	N–S	S–N	Elevation	Latitude, Longitude	Description
2.05	29.8	192.4	8,890'	37.82129°N, 119.27635°W	site for 6+ tents on open flat with scattered lodgepole pine to east of the trail (toward river)
2.06	29.9	192.3	8,900'	37.82045°N, 119.27551°W	space for 3 tents in small lodgepole pine flat west of the trail
2.07	30.6	191.6	8,910'	37.81224°N, 119.26884°W	space for 3 tents on a knob southwest of the trail (37.81182°N, 119.26873°W)
2.08	31.8	190.4	8,970'	37.79687°N, 119.26229°W	space for 3 tents beneath lodgepole pines to the west of trail; additional smaller sites nearby; views to Mounts Lyell and Maclure from adjacent meadow
2.09	32.1	190.1	8,970'	37.79387°N, 119.26275°W	space for 4–6 tents under lodgepole pine cover to the west of trail
2.10	32.3	189.9	9,000'	37.79085°N, 119.26167°W	historic Lyell Forks campsite, with giant lodgepole-pine log wedges as camp tables; site is right at the forest–meadow boundary with lovely views; 4+ tent sites (37.79085°N, 119.26006°W)
2.11	32.4	189.8	9,070'	37.78889°N, 119.26273°W	large area on flat shelf to the north of the trail; continue well over 100' from the trail for the best sites
2.12 🐻	33.4	188.8	9,680'	37.77910°N, 119.26294°W	head southwest to a flat shaded by lodgepole pines with space for 4+ tents; slightly north of the Upper Lyell bridge
2.13 🐻	33.5	188.7	9,660'	37.77776°N, 119.26237°W	from the west side of the Upper Lyell bridge, head southwest to reach a cluster of about 4 tent sites in lodgepole pine forest
2.14 🐻	33.5	188.7	9,650'	37.77765°N, 119.26200°W	from the southeastern side of the Upper Lyell bridge follow a spur trail downstream, passing sites for 6+ tents; options continue for 500'
2.15 🐻	34.4	187.8	10,200'	37.76807°N, 119.25648°W	sites for many tents to the east of the trail beneath tall multistemmed whitebark pine and a few lodgepole pines; continue northeast along the ridge for additional options
2.16 🐻	35.0	187.2	10,510'	37.76192°N, 119.25811°W	use trail ascending the Lyell Fork Tuolumne toward Mount Lyell departs south from here; explore to find scattered small, sandy patches among slabs
3.01 🐻	37.6	184.6	10,390'	37.76144°N, 119.23084°W	site coordinates do not refer to an exact site but an invitation to explore north, including to the north of the creek; it is relatively flat here, with somewhat less vegetation than lower down; if you camp near here, be very aware of your toileting choice, avoiding perennial and seasonal water channels; do not camp on vegetation; beautiful landscape of meadows and scattered whitebark pines
3.02 🐻	38.4	183.8	10,150'	37.75481°N, 119.22351°W	several sandy single-tent sites on slab with scattered whitebark pine to the east of the trail; explore farther east for more options, ensuring you are 100' from water
3.03 🐻	38.8	183.4	10,080'	37.75103°N, 119.22041°W	several sandy single-tent sites among slabs with scattered trees to the east of the trail
3.04 🐻	38.9	183.3	10,060'	37.75008°N, 119.22007°W	Rush Creek crossing; site for 4 tents under lodgepole pines east of the trail; additional sites that are more open once across a side creek
3.05 🐻	39.3	182.9	9,880'	37.74696°N, 119.21530°W	space for 2 tents on a sandy shelf east of the trail; expansive views
3.06 🐻	39.7	182.5	9,710'	37.74473°N, 119.21497°W	space for 2–4 tents under lodgepole pine cover to the south of the trail
3.07 🐻	39.8	182.4	9,670'	37.74434°N, 119.21309°W	sandy flats with space for 4–6 tents to the southwest of the trail among slab ribs; view to the top of the crest; good sites after both 100' and 200' (37.74383°N, 119.21362°W)
3.08 🐻	39.8	182.4	9,660'	37.74421°N, 119.21276°W	site in lodgepole pine flat for about 3 tents in the direction of the creek
3.09 🐻	39.0	183.2	9,640'	37.74389°N, 119.21127°W	Rush Creek junction; cross creek and head southeast to site for about 4 tents on a knob under lodgepole pine cover (37.74396°N, 119.21077°W)

Camp ID	N–S	S–N	Elevation	Latitude, Longitude	Description
4.01 ⊗	41.4	180.8	10,230'	37.73655°N, 119.19430°W	Island Pass; selection of about 3 sandy single-tent sites, surrounded by meadows and clusters of whitebark pine; located about 200' west of the trail
4.02 ⊗	41.6	180.6	10,230'	37.73450°N, 119.19256°W	Island Pass; several scattered single-tent sites, mostly near clusters of trees or occasionally in open, sandy flats; east and west of the trail, north and south of the tarns; look around and ensure you are 100' from water
4.03 ⊗	41.8	180.4	10,210'	37.73256°N, 119.19009°W	south of Island Pass; 3 sandy campsites to the south of the trail with good Banner Peak views; no water
4.04 ⊗	43.1	179.1	9,850'	37.72849°N, 119.17130°W	Thousand Island Lake; head west along the use trail around the lake's north shore to sandy patches among slabs and scattered trees; first sites after 0.15 mile (37.72789°N, 119.17547°W), with more and more options the farther you continue (e.g. 37.72781°N, 119.17851°W); camping prohibited within 0.25 mile of the lake's outlet
4.05 ⊗	43.3	178.9	9,840'	37.72713°N, 119.16924°W	Thousand Island Lake; head west along a use trail above the lake's south shore; hunt for open, sandy sites once past the first peninsula (camping is prohibited within 0.25 mile of the lake's outlet and within 100' of water); expect to walk 0.25–0.5 mile to good options
4.06 ⊗	43.6	178.6	9,910'	37.72462°N, 119.16622°W	space for 3–4 tents strewn along ridge west of Emerald Lake under lodgepole and whitebark pines
4.07 ⊗	43.7	178.5	9,910'	37.72389°N, 119.16393°W	Emerald Lake; 6 sandy sites beneath lodgepole pines; do not expand site by camping on grass (37.72424°N, 119.16367°W); additional options along the northeast side of the lake
4.08 ⊗	44.0	178.2	9,950'	37.72190°N, 119.16050°W	Ruby Lake; bench northeast of lake has scattered sites for 6+ tents surrounded by lodgepole and whitebark pine
4.09 ⊗	44.0	178.2	9,920'	37.72150°N, 119.15949°W	Ruby Lake; scattered single-tent sites under hemlocks and on open slab to the southeast of the lake's outlet; there are many illegal campsites near the trail—ensure you are in a legal site, a full 100' from trail and water
4.10 ⊗	44.8	177.4	9,940'	37.71529°N, 119.15660°W	Garnet Lake; head west along a downward-trending use trail that leads to a multitude of campsites along Garnet Lake's north shore; the first site is after 0.25 mile (space for 1–2 small tents on knob above lake (37.72148°N, 119.15953°W)), with far more options after 0.5 mile (e.g. several sandy single-tent sites dispersed across open slab [37.71197°N, 119.16211°W]; long, sandy flat with space for 4+ tents [37.71261°N, 119.16434°W])
4.11 ⊗	46.4	175.8	10,120'	37.70737°N, 119.15067°W	1 quite small site on the top of bluffs; unreliable late-season water
4.12 ⊗	48.0	174.2	9,270'	37.69522°N, 119.14928°W	2 sites, each with space for 2–4 tents under hemlock and lodgepole pine; unreliable late-season water; ensure you are 100' from water (37.69522°N, 119.14984°W; 37.69474°N, 119.14989°W)
4.13 ⊗	48.3	173.9	9,110'	37.69224°N, 119.14602°W	site for 4+ tents between the trail and the creek under a canopy of lodgepole pine, western white pine, and hemlock, and surrounded by small volcanic outcrops; west of the trail; unreliable late-season water
4.14 ⊗	48.5	173.7	9,000'	37.69060°N, 119.14333°W	many open, sandy tent sites scattered along a bluff above the river; just northeast of the Ediza Lake junction
4.15	50.9	171.3	9,340'	37.68799°N, 119.12137°W	Rosalie Lake; many sites for 1–2 tents east of the lake, some shaded by hemlocks and others in open, sandy patches farther east with views to San Joaquin Ridge; options along a 300' distance southeast of the outlet (all legal campsites are east of the trail)
4.16	51.5	170.7	9,590'	37.68311°N, 119.11971°W	Gladys Lake; selection of sites for 1–2 tents in scattered trees or among slabs along the north and northeast shore; sites start 200' east of the trail (37.68337°N, 119.11833°W; 37.68381°N, 119.11845°W)

Camp ID	N–S	S–N	Elevation	Latitude, Longitude	Description
4.17	51.9	170.3	9,680'	37.67952°N, 119.11745°W	head southeast from the trail to sandy sites on shelf with amazing views to Mammoth Mountain and the Silver Divide; no water
4.18	52.5	169.7	9,440'	37.67393°N, 119.11432°W	Trinity Lakes; space for 3–4 tents in forest-ringed opening east of trail; ensure you are 100' from trail and water, as not all tent pads are legal
4.19	52.6	169.6	9,420'	37.67330°N, 119.11276°W	Trinity Lakes; open, sandy sites for several tents 200' east of trail among low slab and scattered trees (37.67381°N, 119.11224°W); more options 500' from trail (37.67421°N, 119.11125°W)
4.20	52.8	169.4	9,330'	37.67111°N, 119.11001°W	Trinity Lakes; head 500' east of trail to sites on a rise in the center of the cluster of lakes (37.67111°N, 119.11001°W); ensure you are 100' from water
4.21	53.6	168.6	9,180'	37.66312°N, 119.10329°W	Trinity Lakes; open, sandy area between the trail and the outlet of the biggest Trinity Lake, with additional options east of the outlet; ensure you are 100' from the trail and water
4.22	56.0	166.2	8,140'	37.64336°N, 119.09631°W	Minaret Creek; about 4 tent sites on knob above the creek; good choice environmentally, but dusty
4.23	56.1	166.1	8,110'	37.64192°N, 119.09621°W	Minaret Creek; small site in open lodgepole pine and red fir forest to the northwest of the Minaret Creek crossing; beautiful cobbled creek
4.24	56.1	166.1	8,100'	37.64152°N, 119.09602°W	Minaret Creek; openings in lodgepole pine and red fir upstream along Minaret Creek's southwest bank
4.25	57.1	165.1	7,690'	37.63292°N, 119.08902°W	Devils Postpile; head south and then east from the northern Devils Postpile junction to the trailhead and first-come, first-served campground (37.63193°N, 119.08548°W) (note: closed since 2016 and future status unknown)
4.26	59.4	162.8	7,650'	37.61110°N, 119.07659°W	Red's Meadow Campground; head north from the Rainbow Falls junction to Red's Meadow Resort and on to the campground; follow the well-traveled trail just northeast of the resort area; $23/campsite; sites A, B, and C reserved for backpackers (also $23; 37.61959°N, 119.07470°W)
4.27	62.2	160.0	8,660'	37.59125°N, 119.05851°W	Lower Crater Meadow; nice site 0.3 mile east between the trail and the creek (37.59281°N, 119.05306°W); head northeast from the Lower Crater Meadow–JMT junction
4.28	62.3	159.9	8,670'	37.59060°N, 119.05826°W	Lower Crater Meadow; head southwest from the trail to scattered sites for 1–2 tents on the lower slopes of the southern Red Cone
4.29	62.4	159.8	8,710'	37.59009°N, 119.05727°W	Big, open lodgepole-pine flat with lots of legal campsites, including well east and south of the waypoint; Crater Creek never far away
4.30	63.1	159.1	8,930'	37.58458°N, 119.05004°W	Upper Crater Meadow; open pumice site with space for about 4 tents between the trail and the creek; ensure you select tent sites that are a full 100' from the trail and creek; additional space for 6+ tents at the northeast side of Upper Crater Meadow, 0.2 mile east of the JMT (37.58511°N, 119.04800°W)
5.01 Ⓧ	64.8	157.4	9,210'	37.56539°N, 119.03931°W	space for 2–3 tents on a flat pumice knob to the west of the trail beneath scattered lodgepole pine; water from nearby springs
5.02 Ⓧ	65.1	157.1	9,110'	37.56377°N, 119.03424°W	Deer Creek; space for 4+ tents on the northwest side of the crossing shaded by mixed conifers; additional sites on the south side; ensure you select sites a full 100' from trail and water

Camp ID	N–S	S–N	Elevation	Latitude, Longitude	Description
5.03 ⊗	70.3	151.9	9,990'	37.53846°N, 118.97274°W	Duck Creek; head downslope (south) from the trail to find small sites under lodgepole pines near the riverbank; parallel creek downstream up to 500' for a selection of sites for 1–2 tents
5.04 ⊗	70.4	151.8	10,040'	37.53905°N, 118.97051°W	Duck Creek; space for 3–4 tents in a small site in trees south of the trail; site not visible from the trail; note most campsites visible both north and south of the trail here are too close to either the trail or water
5.05 ⊗	70.8	151.4	10,360'	37.53636°N, 118.96994°W	space for 2 tents on sandy patches on a ledge to the southeast of the Duck Pass junction; best spots not visible from the trail; no water
5.06 ⊗	72.7	149.5	9,980'	37.52897°N, 118.95029°W	Purple Lake at Ram Lake junction; head along Purple Lake's northwest shore to find a large selection of legal sites, some on a rib after 0.1 mile (37.53024°N, 118.94979°W) and others on the slope above (37.53049°N, 118.95131°W)
5.07 ⊗	72.9	149.3	9,940'	37.52750°N, 118.94951°W	large site along Purple Creek between the trail and creek with space for 4+ tents; 0.2 mile below the Purple Creek–JMT junction (37.52469°N, 118.95150°W)
5.08 ⊗	73.7	148.5	10,390'	37.52302°N, 118.94481°W	small shelves to the south of the trail make good campsites if you get water from the small lake located 140' in elevation below the trail (lake not shown on maps but is permanent)
5.09 ⊗	74.6	147.6	10,400'	37.51615°N, 118.93706°W	Lake Virginia; use trail leads south along the lake's west shore to collection of sites for 10+ tents set back from the lake in clusters of whitebark or lodgepole pine, or in the open (e.g., 37.51409°N, 118.93620°W; 37.51330°N, 118.93700°W); first sites you encounter are a bit sloping, but those farther south are flat; excellent views
5.10 ⊗	74.7	147.5	10,350'	37.51589°N, 118.93481°W	Lake Virginia; a few single-tent sites on knobs sheltered by whitebark pines to the north of the trail
5.11 ⊗	75.3	146.9	10,410'	37.51056°N, 118.93103°W	sandy flats with space for a few tents near Lake Virginia's east shore and satellite tarn; good location to camp if it is windy
5.12 ⊗	76.8	145.4	9,580'	37.50281°N, 118.92278°W	Tully Hole; site for about 4 tents under partial lodgepole pine cover at the eastern edge of Tully Hole (37.50240°N, 118.92032°W); head 0.15 mile east from the lowest switchback corner northeast of the McGee Pass–JMT junction
5.13 ⊗	77.2	145.0	9,510'	37.49901°N, 118.92756°W	Fish Creek; sandy sites for 2+ tents on an open, broad, flat ridge on the south side of the creek (37.49832°N, 118.92653°W); only 0.1 mile from the trail but inaccessible at high water
5.14 ⊗	77.4	144.8	9,400'	37.49618°N, 118.92995°W	Fish Creek; about 3 tent sites under lodgepole pine cover on a bench on the south side of the creek (37.49564°N, 118.92865°W); only 200' from the trail but inaccessible at high water
5.15 ⊗	77.9	144.3	9,220'	37.49228°N, 118.93240°W	site for 3 tents in hemlock and lodgepole pine forest, a bit south of Fish Creek bridge; west of the trail
5.16 ⊗	78.0	144.2	9,190'	37.49143°N, 118.93292°W	site with 3–4 tent pads on an open knob with scattered lodgepole pines just northwest of the Cascade Valley junction; many visible sites are illegal, but there are other options 100–200' from the trail; west of the trail
5.17 ⊗	78.5	143.7	9,520'	37.48749°N, 118.93450°W	site for 4 small tents among heath vegetation, hemlock, and lodgepole pine on a small bench; west of the trail; water in gully below
5.18 ⊗	79.1	143.1	9,760'	37.48134°N, 118.93480°W	site for 4 tents beneath scattered lodgepole pines to the north of the trail; sites south of the trail are illegal
5.19 ⊗	79.4	142.8	9,880'	37.47986°N, 118.93263°W	1–2 tent sites beneath scattered lodgepole pines to southeast of trail; continue to a shallow knob for a few additional single-tent options

Camp ID	N–S	S–N	Elevation	Latitude, Longitude	Description
5.20 ⊗	80.2	142.0	10,290'	37.47772°N, 118.92424°W	Squaw Lake; 2–3 single-tent sites on the slab ridge west of (away from) the lake; there are at most 2 single-tent sites along the lake's north shore that are a full 100' from the trail and water; most campsites here are illegal; open views and evening sun
5.21 ⊗	80.7	141.5	10,570'	37.47429°N, 118.92891°W	head east past a small tarn to scattered, sandy single-tent sites on a bedrock rib with scattered clusters of white-bark pine
5.22 ⊗	80.9	141.3	10,540'	37.47283°N, 118.92816°W	Chief Lake; head south from trail to the west shore of Chief Lake, where there is a selection of sites for 1–2 tents in sandy flats and beneath clusters of whitebark pine (e.g., 37.47090°N, 118.92877°W; 37.46946°N, 118.92956°W); ensure you are 100' from the shore
6.01 ⊗	82.7	139.5	10,440'	37.45732°N, 118.91848°W	Silver Pass Lake; head 0.15–0.2 mile west to a few sandy sites for 1–2 tents beneath clusters of whitebark pine near the southeast lakeshore; many established sites too close to the lake; additional sites on slabs at the lake's southwest corner
6.02 ⊗	84.2	138.0	9,700'	37.44156°N, 118.91944°W	Silver Pass Creek; follow a use trail southwest to lodgepole pine flat with space for 3–4 tents
6.03 ⊗	84.4	137.8	9,640'	37.44125°N, 118.91568°W	cross Silver Pass Creek to reach a selection of large sites shaded by lodgepole pine at the northwest corner of the large meadow; previously popular with stock groups
6.04 ⊗	84.6	137.6	9,640'	37.44026°N, 118.91287°W	cross Silver Pass Creek to reach several sites: at the northern edge of the large meadow, on a bedrock knob within the meadow, and at the meadow's eastern edge; all sites difficult to access during high water
6.05 ⊗	85.6	136.6	8,920'	37.43606°N, 118.90749°W	Pocket Meadow; 3 tent sites in lodgepole pine flat west of the trail; legal location if—and only if—you're camped beneath the trees, not in the surrounding meadow, and are 100' from all water sources
6.06 ⊗	85.8	136.4	8,920'	37.43365°N, 118.90861°W	south end Pocket Meadow; space for 3 tents in lodgepole pine forest between the trail and the creek; additional space for several groups on the far (west) side of North Fork Mono Creek (not accessible at high water)
6.07	86.2	136.0	8,720'	37.42802°N, 118.91031°W	North Fork Mono Creek; 2+ tent sites in a sandy flat among bedrock ribs to the west of the trail
6.08	86.3	135.9	8,700'	37.42682°N, 118.90983°W	North Fork Mono Creek; 6+ tent sites on a broad, sandy flat among scattered juniper, Jeffrey pine, and lodgepole pine; river now 0.1 mile to the west, with more sites as you approach it
6.09	86.9	135.3	8,320'	37.42098°N, 118.91107°W	site for 3–4 tents in open Jeffrey pine forest to the south of the trail; first tent sites are too close to the trail, but there are additional sites farther back
6.10	87.6	134.6	7,980'	37.41550°N, 118.91512°W	Mono Creek; sites for several groups between the trail and Mono Creek (to the south), with some sites in white fir forest and others on slab; only use sites a full 100' from the trail and water
6.11	88.3	133.9	7,890'	37.41219°N, 118.92350°W	north bank Mono Creek; head east from the trail, paralleling the creek upstream, across open flats with slab ribs and scattered Jeffrey pines and junipers; there are sites for 10+ tents scattered across a distance of 0.25 mile
6.12	88.4	133.8	7,880'	37.41110°N, 118.92461°W	Mono Creek; 3 tent pads in open, sandy sites between the trail and the creek
6.13	93.6	128.6	9,440'	37.37856°N, 118.90607°W	3+ flat, sandy expanses below the trail; excellent views and beautiful junipers; water 0.4 mile up the trail at a reliable spring or 0.1 mile down the trail at an ephemeral stream (37.37828°N, 118.90617°W)

Camp ID	N–S	S–N	Elevation	Latitude, Longitude	Description
6.14	94.2	128.0	9,170'	37.37690°N, 118.90263°W	head downslope from the trail to sandy flats on knob, although tent pads slightly sloping; 1–2 tent pads; no water by midsummer; there is a good option 0.25 mile down the ridge from which you could connect to the Bear Creek Trail
6.15	94.8	127.4	9,000'	37.37167°N, 118.89507°W	2–3 sandy tent pads among bedrock slabs to the west of the trail; open views
6.16	95.2	127.0	8,950'	37.36820°N, 118.88851°W	head west along the Bear Creek Trail, reaching a large site (6+ tents) under lodgepole pine cover after 0.1 mile (37.36829°N, 118.88992°W) and additional sites for 4+ tents on benches above Bear Creek after 0.6 mile (37.36988°N, 118.89784°W); other options as well; very limited camping for the next 2 miles southbound along the JMT
6.17	96.3	125.9	9,160'	37.35600°N, 118.87937°W	space for 2 tents on a bench shaded by lodgepole pine; head east from trail, away from Bear Creek; ensure you select a legal site, as several tent pads are too close to the trail
6.18	97.1	125.1	9,280'	37.34690°N, 118.87816°W	site for 2 tents on the east side of the trail beneath lodgepole pines
6.19	97.5	124.7	9,380'	37.34291°N, 118.87323°W	3 sandy single-tent sites among slab between the trail and the creek; ensure you are 100' from trail and water
6.20	98.4	123.8	9,580'	37.33126°N, 118.86687°W	Bear Creek crossing; 2 small, sandy single-tent sites at the border of forest and expansive slabs; head west from trail
6.21	98.5	123.7	9,580'	37.33065°N, 118.86678°W	Bear Creek crossing; space for 4–6 tents in sandy patches to the east and southeast of the Seven Gables Lakes (East Fork Bear Creek) junction
6.22 ⊗	99.6	122.6	10,020'	37.31941°N, 118.86958°W	Rosemarie Meadow; several sites, each for 1–2 tents, on the low knob east of the trail; ensure you select sites 100' from the trail
6.23 ⊗	99.9	122.3	10,040'	37.31665°N, 118.87215°W	Rosemarie Meadow; various sites at (and beyond) the meadow's perimeter, including sites to the east and southwest and a large site a short distance along the Rose Lake Trail
6.24 ⊗	100.9	121.3	10,410'	37.30418°N, 118.87459°W	Marshall Lake; 2–3 tent pads on a sandy flat below the trail toward the lake; area around Marshall Lake quite bouldery and rough despite appearing flat on a map, thus few camping options
6.25 ⊗	101.2	121.0	10,550'	37.30167°N, 118.87148°W	Marie Lake; 5 small single-tent sites in sandy patches among slab or atop slab to the northeast of the outlet; ensure you are 100' from all water sources to camp
6.26 ⊗	101.5	120.7	10,570'	37.29853°N, 118.87150°W	Marie Lake; area with space for 6+ tents, spread across many small sandy sites to the west of the trail (away from the lake) among whitebark pine
7.01 ⊗	103.2	119.0	10,540'	37.28078°N, 118.87487°W	Heart Lake; space for 2 tents on open slabs west of the lake's outlet
7.02 ⊗	104.0	118.2	10,210'	37.27255°N, 118.87534°W	Sallie Keyes Lakes; 2 openings in lodgepole pine forest between the 2 upper lakes, each with space for 2–3 tents; head west from trail
7.03 ⊗	104.2	118.0	10,200'	37.27051°N, 118.87623°W	middle Sallie Keyes Lake; site for about 4 tents beneath lodgepole pine cover; head north from the outlet
7.04 ⊗	104.5	117.7	10,190'	37.26653°N, 118.87730°W	lower Sallie Keyes Lake; expansive, flat, open lodgepole pine forest east of the trail with space for many tents; near the old snow-survey cabin
7.05 ⊗	105.1	117.1	10,010'	37.26068°N, 118.87439°W	space for 4+ tents in sandy flat beneath scattered lodgepole pines; water usually available in nearby meadow
7.06	106.4	115.8	9,760'	37.25410°N, 118.86494°W	Senger Creek; head 400' east (37.25466°N, 118.86389°W) or 400' west (37.25361°N, 118.86612°W) along the north bank of Senger Creek to reach large sites ringed by lodgepole pines; each holds 4–6 tents

Camp ID	N–S	S–N	Elevation	Latitude, Longitude	Description
7.07 🐾	110.3	111.9	7,800'	37.23714°N, 118.87769°W	Blayney Meadows–Muir Trail Ranch area; continue toward the river from the Muir Trail Ranch resupply station; there are a few sites beneath scattered juniper and aspens on the slopes north of the South Fork San Joaquin River (37.23486°N, 118.88012°W); when water levels are low, there are additional sites south of the river; absolutely ensure you are 100' from water in this highly impacted area
7.08 🐾	110.3	111.9	7,840'	37.22587°N, 118.86357°W	head 250' south to expansive flats on a knob above the South Fork San Joaquin (37.22455°N, 118.86358°W); one of the first easily accessed big, legal sites east of Muir Trail Ranch
7.09	111.1	111.1	7,990'	37.22268°N, 118.84850°W	follow a use trail 0.1 mile south to a large (6+-tent) riverside campsite on a terrace shaded by Jeffrey pines (37.22103°N, 118.84646°W); secluded, beautiful location
7.10	111.8	110.4	8,030'	37.22367°N, 118.83878°W	head about 400' south (toward the river) to a selection of sandy flats beneath Jeffrey and lodgepole pines
7.11	112.1	110.1	8,090'	37.22525°N, 118.83290°W	Piute Creek bridge; 3 tent pads on open bench beneath Jeffrey pines northeast of the bridge
7.12	112.2	110.0	8,080'	37.22490°N, 118.83248°W	Piute Creek bridge; spaces for 4+ tents in openings beneath junipers, Jeffrey pines, and white firs; head west from the trail
7.13	112.3	109.9	8,060'	37.22371°N, 118.83005°W	space for 6+ tents on lodgepole pine flat along the river; head west from trail; do not use sites within 25' of water, and do not establish new sites here
7.14	112.6	109.6	8,100'	37.22174°N, 118.82700°W	4 tent pads on a sandy shelf above the river; head west from trail; do not establish new sites here
7.15	113.6	108.6	8,230'	37.21350°N, 118.81625°W	Aspen Meadow; sandy, open spot with space for 2 tents; just west of the trail
7.16	113.7	108.5	8,240'	37.21257°N, 118.81418°W	Aspen Meadow; room for 2 tents on a shelf shaded by lodgepole pine above the river; head west from the trail; ensure you are camped 25' from water, and do not establish new sites here
7.17	114.8	107.4	8,380'	37.20301°N, 118.80094°W	expansive area beneath lodgepole pine–red fir cover that can accommodate several groups (about 8 tents total); head north from the southwest side of the bridge
7.18	115.0	107.2	8,430'	37.20093°N, 118.79911°W	space for 3–4 tents in an opening ringed by lodgepole pines; just east of the trail
7.19	115.6	106.6	8,480'	37.19344°N, 118.79565°W	Goddard Canyon junction; large flat beneath scattered lodgepole pines west (uphill) of the trail
7.20	115.7	106.5	8,480'	37.19286°N, 118.79477°W	Goddard Canyon junction; space for about 6 tents in open, sandy flats southeast of the bridge
7.21	115.9	106.3	8,480'	37.19561°N, 118.79489°W	4 tent sites in opening under lodgepole pine cover at the base of the switchbacks to Evolution Valley
7.22	117.1	105.1	9,200'	37.19516°N, 118.78420°W	small, sandy spots for 3–4 tents on a bluff above the trail; head south on a steep use trail
7.23	117.5	104.7	9,240'	37.19679°N, 118.77995°W	Evolution Valley; site for 2 tents on a bench shaded by lodgepole pine; between trail and river
7.24	117.6	104.6	9,250'	37.19679°N, 118.77796°W	Evolution Meadow; large opening ringed by lodgepole pines (stock camp); between trail and river
7.25	117.9	104.3	9,240'	37.19585°N, 118.77347°W	Evolution Meadow; sites for 3 tents in opening between the trail and meadow
7.26	118.8	103.4	9,480'	37.19121°N, 118.75980°W	2–3 tent sites in sandy openings among dry meadows; between trail and river
7.27	119.4	102.8	9,560'	37.18882°N, 118.75158°W	site for 3 tents in lodgepole pine flat above the river
7.28	119.7	102.5	9,640'	37.18837°N, 118.74641°W	McClure Meadow; 3 tent sites on open slab between the trail and meadow; scattered lodgepole pine in fractures

Camp ID	N–S	S–N	Elevation	Latitude, Longitude	Description
7.29	119.8	102.4	9,640'	37.18825°N, 118.74574°W	McClure Meadow; flats shaded by lodgepole pine; can accommodate 4–6 tents, spread along the trail across several hundred feet; beautiful views to Mount Darwin and the Hermit
7.30	120.0	102.2	9,650'	37.18784°N, 118.74158°W	eastern end of McClure Meadow; several small to large sites shaded by lodgepole pine; beautiful views to Mount Darwin and the Hermit
7.31	120.5	101.7	9,680'	37.18542°N, 118.73447°W	2–3 tent sites in opening in lodgepole pine forest; stretch of river with pools and small cascades
7.32	120.7	101.5	9,740'	37.18425°N, 118.73097°W	Colby Meadow; sites for many tents, some in a large flat shaded by lodgepole pine and others in sandy openings between slabs; between the trail and river
7.33	122.0	100.2	9,950'	37.17468°N, 118.71439°W	west side Darwin Canyon drainage crossing; sites on sand and slab for about 3 tents; views to the Hermit; between trail and Evolution Creek
7.34	122.1	100.1	9,940'	37.17380°N, 118.71369°W	follow the use trail 400' south (toward Evolution Creek) to a site for 4–6 tents in a big lodgepole pine flat (37.17286°N, 118.71443°W)
7.35 🚫	123.9	98.3	10,870'	37.17215°N, 118.70030°W	Evolution Lake; with searching you can find 8+ low-impact tent sites within 400' of this location, all small sites on sand or slab, usually near stunted whitebark pines; look on the slab rib to the north, the knob to the west, and the flat slabs to the south
7.36 🚫	125.9	96.3	10,980'	37.15250°N, 118.69541°W	Sapphire Lake; while there are a few campsites near the trail, there are many more options along the east side of the lake, especially on a shelf above the outlet tarns (37.15327°N, 118.69351°W) and halfway around the east shore on slabs and sand (37.14948°N, 118.69243°W); simply ensure you are 100' from water and aren't camping on any plants
7.37 🚫	127.8	94.4	11,430'	37.12875°N, 118.69734°W	Wanda Lake; space for about 5 small tents, distributed over a large area near the outlet and up to 300' south along Wanda's shore; each site is small, sandy, and surrounded by slabs; beautiful views; do not establish new sites here
7.38 🚫	128.5	93.7	11,480'	37.12195°N, 118.68829°W	Wanda Lake; space for 2 tents on the shallow ridge that separates the trail from the lake; lovely views of Wanda Lake and to Mount Goddard
8.01 🚫	130.4	91.8	11,700'	37.11410°N, 118.66521°W	sandy site for 1–2 tents among slabs next to a small tarn above Helen Lake (37.11474°N, 118.66553°W); head 200' northwest from the trail
8.02 🚫	132.0	90.2	11,130'	37.12380°N, 118.64954°W	space for 3 tents in sandy patch on a knob, sheltered by tall whitebark pines
8.03 🚫	132.9	89.3	10,830'	37.12162°N, 118.64148°W	space for 4–6 tents on the shelf east of the creek beneath whitebark pines
8.04 🚫	133.1	89.1	10,700'	37.11945°N, 118.64131°W	2 tent sites in small opening beneath whitebark pines just east of the trail, and more options if you explore farther east
8.05 🚫	133.2	89.0	10,660'	37.11823°N, 118.63990°W	single-tent site under lodgepole pines to the west of the trail; good views to the Black Giant
8.06 🚫	133.5	88.7	10,480'	37.11608°N, 118.63964°W	space for about 5 tents on a lodgepole pine flat west of the trail; good views to the Black Giant
8.07 🚫	133.9	88.3	10,330'	37.11434°N, 118.63713°W	Starr Camp; 4+ tent sites among encroaching young lodgepole and whitebark pines to the south of the trail; beautiful views of Langille Peak, the Black Giant, and Le Conte Canyon
8.08 🚫	134.6	87.6	9,870'	37.11338°N, 118.62948°W	space for about 4 tents under hemlock, lodgepole, and whitebark pine cover to the south of the trail; lots of little patches for tents among trees, just above the NO FIRES sign

Camp ID	N–S	S–N	Elevation	Latitude, Longitude	Description
8.09	135.1	87.1	9,490'	37.11259°N, 118.62126°W	Rock Monster; sites for 5 tents in partially shaded flats south of the trail
8.10	135.8	86.4	9,310'	37.11359°N, 118.61110°W	space for 4+ tents under lodgepole pine cover between the trail and river
8.11	136.1	86.1	9,260'	37.11280°N, 118.60627°W	Big Pete Meadow; space for 4+ tents, spread across several small sites under lodgepole pine cover to either side of the trail; just east of creek crossing
8.12	136.3	85.9	9,250'	37.11101°N, 118.60385°W	Big Pete Meadow; a lateral trail leads 300' west to a large opening under lodgepole pine cover (37.11081°N, 118.60489°W); more options nearby
8.13	136.7	85.5	9,010'	37.10620°N, 118.60095°W	space for 1–2 tents on a sandy shelf west of the trail; excellent views of Langille Peak and down Le Conte Canyon
8.14	137.1	85.1	8,880'	37.10222°N, 118.59844°W	Little Pete Meadow; stock camp under lodgepole pines at edge of meadow; additional options just to the north for smaller groups
8.15	137.7	84.5	8,800'	37.09551°N, 118.59478°W	Le Conte Canyon; head southwest to find space for about 3 tents in a stand of lodgepole pine; other options nearby on a shelf above the creek
8.16	137.8	84.4	8,750'	37.09415°N, 118.59432°W	Le Conte Canyon; 2 sites in sandy flats among slabs with good views; walk one switchback up the Bishop Pass Trail, then head south (37.09378°N, 118.59382°W)
8.17	137.8	84.4	8,730'	37.09368°N, 118.59422°W	Le Conte Canyon; space for 5+ tents west of the trail under lodgepole pines; more options 200' to the south
8.18	138.0	84.2	8,690'	37.09118°N, 118.59430°W	Le Conte Canyon; space for 3 tents under lodgepole pines; head east from trail
8.19	138.2	84.0	8,650'	37.08807°N, 118.59503°W	Le Conte Canyon; 5 small tent pads spread across both sides of the trail under lodgepole pines; views to the Citadel; absolutely ensure you are 25' from trail and water, and do not establish new sites here
8.20	139.2	83.0	8,350'	37.07571°N, 118.59661°W	Le Conte Canyon; space for 3 tents on open bench above river; head west from trail; views to Ladder Falls and the Citadel
8.21	139.2	83.0	8,340'	37.07488°N, 118.59638°W	2 sites at edge of sagebrush flat shaded by lodgepole pine between the trail and the river; views to Ladder Falls and the Citadel
8.22	139.4	82.8	8,320'	37.07286°N, 118.59559°W	space for about 3 tents on a river terrace shaded by lodgepole pine; head west from the trail
8.23	140.2	82.0	8,240'	37.06362°N, 118.58920°W	Grouse Meadow; space for 5 tents in a stand of lodgepole pine just west of the trail; do not camp in the meadow
8.24	140.3	81.9	8,250'	37.06302°N, 118.58830°W	Grouse Meadow; space for 3 tents in a stand of lodgepole pine just west of the trail; do not camp in the meadow
8.25	141.1	81.1	8,090'	37.05296°N, 118.58052°W	2 tent sites on a sandy shelf above the Middle Fork Kings; open views
8.26	141.2	81.0	8,040'	37.05285°N, 118.57938°W	space for about 6 tents in a large flat beneath Jeffrey pines at the Middle Fork Trail junction; head south from trail
8.27	141.8	80.4	8,270'	37.05389°N, 118.57064°W	about 3 tent sites on a shelf under lodgepole pine between the trail and the river; nice spot
8.28	142.3	79.9	8,430'	37.05294°N, 118.56344°W	2 tent sites on a shelf above the creek, beneath scattered lodgepole pine cover; head south from trail
8.29	142.5	79.7	8,430'	37.05285°N, 118.56081°W	2 small tent sites under Jeffrey pines; head north from trail
8.30	143.9	78.3	8,680'	37.05359°N, 118.53754°W	space for 4+ tents on lodgepole pine flat between trail and river; pocket of surviving trees
8.31	144.2	78.0	8,730'	37.05486°N, 118.53377°W	space for 3-4 tents in lodgepole pine flat between trail and river; pocket of surviving trees
8.32	144.7	77.5	8,860'	37.05586°N, 118.52628°W	Deer Meadow; expansive flat in lodgepole pine forest that offers dispersed sites for about 12 tents; head toward Palisade Creek (south of trail)

Camp ID	N–S	S–N	Elevation	Latitude, Longitude	Description
8.33	145.2	77.0	8,890'	37.05457°N, 118.51911°W	space for 5 tents in open lodgepole pine and red fir stand just east of the Glacier Creek crossing; head south from trail; a second smaller site 0.1 mile east
8.34	145.4	76.8	8,960'	37.05484°N, 118.51637°W	space for 2–3 tents near the base of the Golden Staircase, shaded by lodgepole pine and red fir; head south from trail
8.35	145.4	76.8	8,980'	37.05466°N, 118.51503°W	space for 2–3 tents near the base of the Golden Staircase, shaded by lodgepole pine and red fir; nice spot; head south from trail
8.36 Ⓧ	147.6	74.6	10,350'	37.05513°N, 118.49596°W	space for 1–2 tents on sandy flat next to hemlocks; head southeast from trail; good views to west
8.37 Ⓧ	148.3	73.9	10,610'	37.06021°N, 118.48894°W	Lower Palisade Lake; there are at least 15 small tent pads within 0.1 mile of this waypoint, scattered to either side of the trail, including across Palisade Creek; the sites are generally in clusters of 1–2 tent pads in sandy nooks among slab; views to the Middle Palisade group
8.38 Ⓧ	149.2	73.0	10,810'	37.05649°N, 118.47655°W	2 sandy sites under whitebark pines; head south from trail; additional options southeast along the trail
8.39 Ⓧ	149.5	72.7	10,850'	37.05455°N, 118.47310°W	space for about 6 tents, each a sandy single-tent site surrounded by whitebark pines, but sites clustered together somewhat; a few more options 200' to the south and downslope toward Upper Palisade Lake; all overlooking Upper Palisade Lake; excellent views; water from a creek a short distance south along the trail
8.40 Ⓧ	149.7	72.5	10,860'	37.05232°N, 118.47135°W	space for 3 tents beneath stunted whitebark pines and overlooking Upper Palisade Lake; excellent views; head west of trail
8.41 Ⓧ	150.2	72.0	10,980'	37.04659°N, 118.46817°W	3 small tent sites under the highest whitebark pines; amazing views down to the Palisade Lakes
9.01 Ⓧ	153.1	69.1	11,620'	37.02904°N, 118.45437°W	Upper Basin; head due east to reach a large lake with 4+ flat, sandy tent sites; broad, open views
9.02 Ⓧ	153.6	68.6	11,500'	37.02338°N, 118.45711°W	Upper Basin; wander in any direction to find sandy tent sites near the many tarns in Upper Basin; make sure you camp on unvegetated areas 100' from water
9.03 Ⓧ	154.9	67.3	11,020'	37.00677°N, 118.45494°W	sandy flats to either side of the trail beneath whitebark pine, each with space for 2 tents; other options farther from the trail
9.04 Ⓧ	155.2	67.0	10,920'	37.00290°N, 118.45314°W	several single-tent sites beneath whitebark pine to the east of the trail
9.05 Ⓧ	156.4	65.8	10,540'	36.98742°N, 118.44801°W	2 sandy tent pads on open slab between the trail and creek; east of the trail
9.06 Ⓧ	157.3	64.9	10,250'	36.97609°N, 118.44262°W	space for 3 tents on a flat with scattered lodgepole pine between the trail and the creek
9.07 Ⓧ	157.4	64.8	10,190'	36.97481°N, 118.44257°W	site for 5 tents in open flat beneath scattered lodgepole pine just east of trail
9.08 Ⓧ	157.4	64.8	10,180'	36.97434°N, 118.44281°W	from cairn marking abandoned trail to Taboose Pass, head east to creek; here there is a large opening under lodgepole pine
9.09 Ⓧ	157.7	64.5	10,050'	36.97025°N, 118.44445°W	south side South Fork Kings crossing; site for 1–2 tents in open lodgepole pine forest; head east from trail
9.10 Ⓧ	157.8	64.4	10,060'	36.96971°N, 118.44430°W	south side South Fork Kings crossing; space for about 5 tents in sandy openings to the west of the trail
9.11 Ⓧ	159.2	63.0	10,860'	36.95873°N, 118.43686°W	2–3 small tent sites spread across both sides of the trail
9.12 Ⓧ	159.4	62.8	10,970'	36.95588°N, 118.43655°W	2 sites, each with room for 2–3 tents, beneath clusters of tall whitebark pine on knobs west of the trail (36.95604°N, 118.43715°W; 36.95616°N, 118.43749°W)
9.13 Ⓧ	159.6	62.6	11,000'	36.95452°N, 118.43531°W	scattered single-tent sites on a small rise with whitebark pines, toward a tarn

Camp ID	N–S	S–N	Elevation	Latitude, Longitude	Description
9.14 ⊗	159.9	62.3	11,040'	36.95091°N, 118.43315°W	Lake Marjorie tarns; 5+ individual tent sites in sandy spots among slabs and whitebark pines between 2 small lakes
9.15 ⊗	160.3	61.9	11,140'	36.94681°N, 118.43176°W	Lake Marjorie; 6+ sandy tent pads within 300' of this way-point; in clusters of 1–2 pads and spread across both sides of the trail
9.16 ⊗	160.4	61.8	11,170'	36.94658°N, 118.42984°W	Lake Marjorie; about 3 sandy tent pads east of the trail; landscape of slabs and whitebark pines
9.17 ⊗	160.8	61.4	11,290'	36.94334°N, 118.42580°W	1–2 sandy spots on slab west of the trail; water a short walk down the trail
10.01 ⊗	163.7	58.5	11,380'	36.92647°N, 118.39954°W	head 500' north to the chain of small lakes; hunt for sandy flats among whitebark pines while still on the JMT with its good vantage point, ensuring you pick a previously impacted location
10.02 ⊗	164.6	57.6	11,020'	36.91751°N, 118.39401°W	4+ sandy tent sites on an open bench 400' east of the trail, with endless options if you explore the expanse of sand and slab beyond
10.03 ⊗	164.9	57.3	10,900'	36.91405°N, 118.39590°W	space for 4+ tents dispersed along the crest of a sandy moraine rib, surrounded by lodgepole pines; head south-east from the trail (away from the lake); highest-elevation campsite near the trail on the south side of Pinchot Pass
10.04 ⊗	165.4	56.8	10,610'	36.90839°N, 118.39822°W	Twin Lakes; selection of sites along the north shore of the lower lake, including space for 2 tents under lodgepole pines after 300' (36.90816°N, 118.39723°W) and 3+ sandy tent pads near the lake's inlet (36.91051°N, 118.39419°W)
10.05 ⊗	165.9	56.3	10,370'	36.90262°N, 118.40042°W	Sawmill Pass junction; small site east of the creek crossing, under lodgepole pine cover
10.06	166.0	56.2	10,280'	36.90185°N, 118.40252°W	4 tent pads on a knob with lodgepole and whitebark pines, just south of the creek crossing
10.07	166.7	55.5	9,800'	36.89931°N, 118.41085°W	space for 10+ tents on a broad shelf shaded by lodgepole pines; head south and east from the trail
10.08	167.9	54.3	9,250'	36.88898°N, 118.42105°W	about 5 tent pads, spread out on a long bench above river; partially shaded by lodgepole pines; head south from trail
10.09	169.7	52.5	8,540'	36.87340°N, 118.43762°W	Woods Creek crossing; large site with room for about 15 tents on the east side of the trail just south of bridge; food-storage box; continuing southeast, there are additional single-tent sites nestled in the forest
10.10	172.0	50.2	9,470'	36.85222°N, 118.41392°W	space for about 5 tents in pads spread across both sides of the trail under lodgepole pine cover; take care not to camp under dead trees
10.11 ⊗	173.6	48.6	10,220'	36.83464°N, 118.40813°W	Dollar Lake; space for 2–4 tents along the north shore and across the South Fork Woods Creek; beautiful reflections of Fin Dome in the lake; camping is prohibited along Dollar Lake's west shore
10.12 ⊗	174.2	48.0	10,310'	36.82765°N, 118.40965°W	Arrowhead Lake; space for about 15 tents; first tent sites are beneath lodgepole pines near where you leave the trail; continue south, paralleling the lakeshore for up to 500' for many more options, both under forest cover and in sandy flats; fantastic view of Fin Dome; food-storage box
10.13 ⊗	175.1	47.1	10,570'	36.81549°N, 118.40548°W	Lower Rae Lake; bench with about 6 sandy tent pads under sparse lodgepole and whitebark pine cover
10.14 ⊗	175.2	47.0	10,580'	36.81487°N, 118.40503°W	Lower Rae Lake; space for 8+ tents on bench with large sandy flats and sparse lodgepole and whitebark pine cover; food-storage box
10.15 ⊗	176.0	46.2	10,600'	36.80638°N, 118.39796°W	Middle Rae Lake; space for about 10 tents on sandy flats among scattered whitebark pines; head 500' west on a spur trail toward lake (36.80691°N, 118.39942°W); food-storage boxes

Camp ID	N–S	S–N	Elevation	Latitude, Longitude	Description
10.16 🅧	176.4	45.8	10,560'	36.80376°N, 118.40133°W	Upper Rae Lake; about 4 scattered single-tent sites on the peninsula between the upper and middle lakes; only use established sites
10.17 🅧	176.6	45.6	10,560'	36.80276°N, 118.40253°W	Upper Rae Lake; about 5 small sandy spots, each for a single tent, among slabs and whitebark pines scattered around the Sixty Lake Basin junction; most sites are not visible from the trail; fantastic views of the Painted Lady and Upper Rae Lake; use only established sites
10.18 🅧	177.3	44.9	11,090'	36.79753°N, 118.40670°W	space for 2–3 tents in a cluster of whitebark pines on a knob with a tarn behind; head northwest from trail
10.19 🅧	177.7	44.5	11,380'	36.79347°N, 118.40945°W	tiny, exposed, single-tent alpine sites in sandy patches between slabs near tarns to west of trail; sites best seen when you are slightly above them
11.01 🅧	179.0	43.2	11,570'	36.78638°N, 118.41346°W	2 small tent pads among whitebark pines near the lake's outlet; head east from trail
11.02 🅧	179.6	42.6	11,080'	36.78453°N, 118.42154°W	2–3 small sandy tent pads near stunted whitebark pines; usually reliable water 400' to east in trailside tarns
11.03 🅧	180.8	41.4	10,750'	36.77065°N, 118.41627°W	Charlotte Lake; large site with space for 10+ tents at the north end of the lake, 0.9 mile off the JMT (36.77810°N, 118.42737°W); additional smaller sites along the lake's east shore; food-storage box; ranger cabin
11.04 🅧	181.2	41.0	10,530'	36.76819°N, 118.41146°W	Bullfrog and Kearsarge Lakes junction; about 5 small tent pads, both northeast and southeast of the junction, among streamside vegetation and foxtail pines; ensure you select one of the sites that is at least 25' from the trail and water
11.05 🅧	181.4	40.8	10,370'	36.76606°N, 118.41086°W	site for a few tents on shelf above creek, with lodgepole pine cover and wet heath vegetation; head south from trail
11.06 🅧	181.8	40.4	10,070'	36.76437°N, 118.40804°W	2–3 tent sites shaded by lodgepole pines to the west of the creek crossing; head south from trail
11.07	182.4	39.8	9,560'	36.76029°N, 118.41194°W	Lower Vidette Meadow; site for 6+ tents in a large opening in lush lodgepole pine forest just upstream of Bubbs Creek junction; head south from trail
11.08	182.7	39.5	9,530'	36.75950°N, 118.40784°W	2 spots next to trail in dry lodgepole pine forest; just north of Vidette Meadow
11.09	182.8	39.4	9,550'	36.75910°N, 118.40618°W	Vidette Meadow; several large sites together accommodate about 10 tents in openings in dry lodgepole pine forest at meadow's edge; views to East Vidette; food-storage box
11.10	182.8	39.4	9,560'	36.75843°N, 118.40501°W	Vidette Meadow; site for about 6 tents in large opening in dry lodgepole pine forest at meadow's edge; views to East Vidette; more options 200' south
11.11	183.6	38.6	9,910'	36.75295°N, 118.39431°W	Upper Vidette Meadow; space for about 10 tents in a large opening in flat lodgepole pine forest; food-storage box; additional option 300' to the south
11.12 🅧	183.8	38.4	9,970'	36.75250°N, 118.39187°W	site for 4–6 tents in dry lodgepole pine forest; head west from trail
11.13 🅧	185.2	37.0	10,400'	36.73781°N, 118.37909°W	space for 4 tents on a shelf between the trail and stream; under lodgepole and whitebark pine cover; a few additional sites 300' to the south
11.14 🅧	185.8	36.4	10,480'	36.73411°N, 118.37560°W	Center Basin junction; space for 10+ tents, most on a large sand-and-slab bench and a few beneath lodgepole pine cover; head west from trail; food-storage box
11.15 🅧	185.8	36.4	10,540'	36.73081°N, 118.37290°W	Bubbs Creek crossing (Center Basin outflow), sites for about 6 tents in lodgepole pine forest just southwest of the creek
11.16 🅧	186.7	35.5	10,910'	36.72066°N, 118.37133°W	3–4 small tent sites on small knob with whitebark pines; spectacular views; unreliable late-season water
11.17 🅧	186.8	35.4	10,940'	36.71969°N, 118.37167°W	3–4 small tent sites on flat shelf with scattered whitebark pines above valley; spectacular views; unreliable late-season water

Camp ID	N–S	S–N	Elevation	Latitude, Longitude	Description
11.18 ⓧ	187.3	34.9	11,230'	36.71312°N, 118.37194°W	upper Bubbs camp; about 6 single-tent sites beneath highest stand of whitebark pine; excellent views
11.19 ⓧ	187.4	34.8	11,240'	36.71321°N, 118.37152°W	about 4 small tent pads in sandy flats to the north of the trail and about 2 to the south of the trail, under scattered whitebark pine cover; amazing views
11.20 ⓧ	188.4	33.8	11,760'	36.71069°N, 118.36528°W	2 small sandy tent pads among slabs and boulders near the small tarn to the east of the trail; be sure to keep off alpine plants
11.21 ⓧ	188.6	33.6	11,890'	36.70779°N, 118.36577°W	4 small sandy tent pads among slabs to the west of the trail; exposed alpine perch with expansive views; be sure to keep off alpine plants
11.22 ⓧ	189.3	32.9	12,250'	36.70248°N, 118.36868°W	Lake 12,258; 2 exposed tent sites overlooking the lake and surrounded by talus; excellent views to Junction Peak; often windy
12.01 ⓧ	191.3	30.9	12,500'	36.69089°N, 118.37425°W	2–3 tiny sandy tent sites among slabs near the outlet of the lake just south of Forester Pass
12.02 ⓧ	192.3	29.9	12,220'	36.67884°N, 118.37960°W	sandy site for 2–3 tents among slabs southeast of the trail, with many additional options southeast and east toward the nearby lakes
12.03 ⓧ	194.4	27.8	11,380'	36.65527°N, 118.38870°W	space for 2 tents beneath lodgepole pine to the east of the trail; seeps with water nearby (occasionally dry)
12.04 ⓧ	195.3	26.9	10,970'	36.64299°N, 118.38745°W	Tyndall Creek crossing; space for 8+ tents in the large sandy opening to the west of the trail; search farther west and south for other options; food-storage box; other options to the northeast, but some locations are a restoration area
12.05 ⓧ	195.6	26.6	10,880'	36.64013°N, 118.38816°W	about 6 tent sites under sparse lodgepole pine shade on a shelf above Tyndall Creek; head west from trail when just north of the Tyndall Creek ranger cabin junction
12.06 ⓧ	196.0	26.2	11,040'	36.63524°N, 118.38553°W	Tyndall Frog Ponds; space for 15+ tents in a large flat close to the trail and then sites strung out along the west shore of the lakes and on the rise to the west; food-storage box
12.07 ⓧ	197.2	25.0	11,440'	36.61927°N, 118.37994°W	Bighorn Plateau; lots of flat, sandy spots along the north side of the lake; no trees or large rocks for shelter; make sure you camp off vegetation and 100' away from the lake
12.08 ⓧ	198.8	23.4	10,800'	36.60135°N, 118.37266°W	site shaded by lodgepole pine with space for 3 tents on a shelf above Wright Creek; head southeast from trail; other, smaller options nearby
12.09 ⓧ	199.0	23.2	10,750'	36.59947°N, 118.37457°W	several sandy sites for 1–2 tents on a shelf with scattered lodgepole pines above Wright Creek; head southeast from trail
12.10 ⓧ	199.2	23.0	10,690'	36.59744°N, 118.37527°W	Wright Creek; a few sites in an opening shaded by lodge-pole pine to the southwest of the creek
12.11 ⓧ	199.8	22.4	10,410'	36.59427°N, 118.37115°W	Wallace Creek north bank; space for about 6 tents to the west (adjacent to a large meadow a short distance along the High Sierra Trail) and space for 4 tents to the east in open lodgepole forest
12.12 ⓧ	199.9	22.3	10,400'	36.59370°N, 118.37078°W	Wallace Creek crossing; space for 6+ tents under scattered lodgepole pines on the southwest side of the crossing; food-storage box
12.13 ⓧ	200.4	21.8	10,650'	36.59103°N, 118.37039°W	1-2 tent sites under lodgepole pines just north of a small creek; head east from trail
12.14 ⓧ	202.0	20.2	10,710'	36.57309°N, 118.37111°W	Sandy Meadow; 2 tent sites at upper edge of the meadow in mixed foxtail–lodgepole pine forest; nearby creeks dry in mid- to late summer
12.15 ⓧ	204.1	18.1	10,710'	36.56478°N, 118.35041°W	Crabtree camping area; head south along the spur trail, immediately passing one expansive flat with space for 10+ tents (36.56465°N, 118.34985°W), then crossing the creek to space for 20+ tents in lodgepole pine forest ringing a meadow (36.56321°N, 118.34908°W); food-storage box; pit toilet; ranger cabin

Camp ID	N–S	S–N	Elevation	Latitude, Longitude	Description
12.16 🐾	206.6	15.6	11,600'	36.57321°N, 118.31608°W	west end Guitar Lake; head south to find sandy sites on the knob north of Guitar Lake and toward the west end of the lake; beautiful views to the Kaweahs and Mount Whitney; no privacy
12.17 🐾	206.8	15.4	11,490'	36.57230°N, 118.31407°W	Guitar Lake; use trail leads south toward the lake's north shore; space for 15+ tents in exposed, sandy sites among slabs; beautiful views to the Kaweahs and Mount Whitney; no privacy
12.18 🐾	206.9	15.3	11,510'	36.57201°N, 118.31267°W	Guitar Lake; space for 10+ tents in small sandy flats among slabs to either side of the trail once east of Arctic Creek; beautiful views to the Kaweahs and Mount Whitney; no privacy
12.19 🐾	207.7	14.5	11,940'	36.56691°N, 118.30349°W	Hitchcock tarns; head up to 0.25 mile west to sheltered sandy flats between the tarns above the Hitchcock Lakes; in early season, there are additional options closer to the trail, both west and south of the waypoint; fantastic views to Mount Whitney
12.20 🐾	209.6	12.6	13,390'	36.56161°N, 118.29345°W	Mount Whitney Trail junction; room for 5 small tents in sandy spots among talus, mostly sheltered by rock walls; amazing views to the west; head east (upslope) from the trail on the switchback just below the Mount Whitney Trail junction; no water
12.21 🐾	211.6	10.6	14,480'	36.57856°N, 118.29218°W	Mount Whitney summit; space for many people in various sandy flats among boulders, although many nooks fit just a sleeping pad, not a tent; views in all directions; often cold and windy; no water
13.01 🐾	216.0	6.2	12,030'	36.56298°N, 118.27914°W	Trail Camp; space for about 20 tents in sandy flats among slabs, on both sides of trail; often cold and windy
13.02 🐾	216.1	6.1	11,980'	36.56337°N, 118.27692°W	head southwest up the gully south of the trail corridor to reach another cluster of sandy tent sites
13.03 🐾	216.2	6.0	11,930'	36.56379°N, 118.27517°W	head north up slabs to a bedrock rib with 5+ sandy nooks among slabs
13.04 🐾	217.4	4.8	11,040'	36.56824°N, 118.26247°W	small open sites on knob; excellent views but far from water
13.05 🐾	217.7	4.5	10,860'	36.56931°N, 118.26222°W	3 tent sites beneath sparse foxtail pine cover on bluffs above Mirror Lake; excellent views but far from water
13.06 🐾	218.4	3.8	10,370'	36.57159°N, 118.25885°W	Outpost Camp; 15+ tents fit in this very large, open, sandy site beneath scattered foxtail pines
13.07 🐾	219.3	2.9	10,030'	36.57499°N, 118.25050°W	Lone Pine Lake; a few small, sandy sites on the rib north of Lone Pine Lake; head east along the spur trail for 0.2 mile to reach the lake (36.57746°N, 118.24730°W)
13.08 🐾	219.4	2.8	10,030'	36.57525°N, 118.25085°W	3 tent sites in lodgepole pine forest to the southwest of the Lone Pine Creek ford

Lateral Trails

This section includes information on the lateral trails diverging from the JMT to trailheads and the main towns adjacent to them. You may need to use these trails for a variety of reasons: to resupply on food, to bail out if a member of your party is sick or injured, or to enter and exit if you are section-hiking the trail.

The trails are organized from north to south according to where they leave the JMT (distance from Happy Isles/Whitney Portal). Each trail summary lists the places, roads, and other trails to which the lateral trail provides access. All GPS coordinates mentioned in the text can be downloaded at tinyurl.com/JMTWaypoints.

Starting on page 84 is a table that includes basic information about each lateral trail, including towns accessed, the length of the trail, elevation gain/loss (starting from the JMT), and distance along the JMT. Also included is the agency in whose jurisdiction the trailhead lies, and the trailhead for which you need to obtain a permit if you are beginning a section hike at this trailhead. (See page 3 for details on how to obtain permits from each park or forest.) Most trail summaries include annotated elevation profiles, displaying trail junctions, major camping areas, and notes about hazards.

Finally, three trail maps are included: one for trails around Lake Edison and Vermilion Valley Resort (see sidebar opposite) and two that accompany the trail summaries for PCT South, from Crabtree to Cottonwood Lakes (page 101) and PCT South, from Crabtree to Cottonwood Pass (page 106).

In general, exiting the JMT for any reason, including resupplying food, becomes more difficult the farther south you are. There are many relatively easy options in the northern third of the trail; a few long but well-graded and well-maintained options in the middle third of the trail (including **Mono Pass, Piute Pass,** and **Bishop Pass** to the east, and **Lake Edison, Bear Creek,** and **Florence Lake** to the west); and only one fairly easy east-side pass south of Bishop Pass: **Kearsarge Pass.** Toward the south, two of the trails heading out to Cedar Grove (Roads End) on the west side, **Woods Creek** and **Bubbs Creek,** are also easy, with virtually no elevation gain (heading west), but keep in mind that the western trailheads are farther from population centers and finding a ride back to your car may prove difficult or expensive since no shuttles service these trailheads.

Not included here are most use trails and routes where the nearest trailhead is more than 20 miles distant. If you know that your route will include considerable time on some of these lateral trails, you may wish to consult other Wilderness Press books, including *Sierra North, Sierra South,* and *Sequoia & Kings Canyon National Parks,* for additional details. *Sierra South* includes trail descriptions and annotated elevation profiles for every lateral trail intersecting the JMT *except* the abandoned trail over Baxter Pass; carrying a digital copy of the book will allow you to easily scheme a plan B once on the trail.

Which Way to Vermilion Valley Resort?

There is much discussion about how to get to and from Vermilion Valley Resort, generally known as VVR, because there are three trails that cross Bear Ridge: the JMT, the Bear Ridge Trail, and the Bear Creek Cutoff Trail. The mileage, elevation gain and loss, and advantages and disadvantages of each route are listed in the table below. Also see the map on the next two pages.

Route	Total Distance (VVR to Bear Creek Junction, in miles)	Total Elevation (VVR to Bear Creek Junction)	Advantages	Disadvantages
Lake Edison Trail + JMT from Mono Creek junction to Bear Creek junction	FERRY: 8.4 (1.4 from ferry wharf to JMT; 7.0 on JMT) WITHOUT FERRY: 13.8 (6.8 from VVR to JMT; 7.0 on JMT)	+2,530'/−1,320' (with ferry) +3,370'/−2,110' (no ferry)	• you walk the entire length of the JMT • beautiful view toward Selden Pass from the top of Bear Ridge • a well-graded, quiet, shady walk	• $24 round-trip for ferry • ferry runs only twice a day (or add 5.4 miles to walk one-way) • climb up Bear Ridge along the JMT can feel very long
Bear Ridge Trail + JMT from Bear Ridge Trail junction to Bear Creek junction	WITH SHUTTLE TO TRAILHEAD: 7.1 (4.8 up the Bear Ridge Trail; 2.3 on JMT) WITHOUT SHUTTLE: 9.4	+2,450'/−1,140' (with shuttle) +2,620'/−1,380' (no shuttle)	• 2 miles shorter than other options • much of the walk is shaded • beautiful view toward Selden Pass from the top of Bear Ridge	• + $10 for ride to trailhead • ride to trailhead offered only twice a day (or add 2.3 miles) • Bear Ridge Trail is not very scenic
Bear Creek Cutoff Trail to Bear Creek–JMT junction	WITH SHUTTLE TO TRAILHEAD: 9.5 WITHOUT SHUTTLE: 12.0	+2,580'/−1,190' (with shuttle) +2,700'/−1,470' (no shuttle)	• truly beautiful walk • follow a spectacular length of river for several miles	• + $10 for ride to trailhead • ride to trailhead offered only twice a day (or add 2.5 miles) • longest route • the distane at lower, hotter elevations

There are also two possible routes from VVR to the Goodale Pass–JMT junction on the north side of Silver Pass: (1) either across Lake Edison and along the Lake Edison Trail to the JMT, then along the JMT over Silver Pass, or (2) leaving the Lake Edison Trail just 1.5 mile from VVR and crossing the Silver Divide via Goodale Pass.

Route	Total Distance (Goodale Pass–JMT junction to VVR, in miles)	Total Elevation (VVR to Goodale Pass–JMT junction)	Advantages	Disadvantages
Silver Pass (along the JMT)	9.1 (with ferry) 14.5 (without ferry)	+3,600'/−700' (with ferry) +4,450'/−1,550' (without ferry)	• follows the actual JMT • shorter distance if the ferry is running	• 2 sometimes-tricky creek crossings • rougher descent (SOBO)
Goodale Pass	11.6	+3,730'/−830'	• shorter distance and less elevation gain if the ferry isn't running • in early summer, avoids 2 potentially difficult stream crossings	• farther from the Sierra Crest and at a lower elevation • more miles through burned terrain

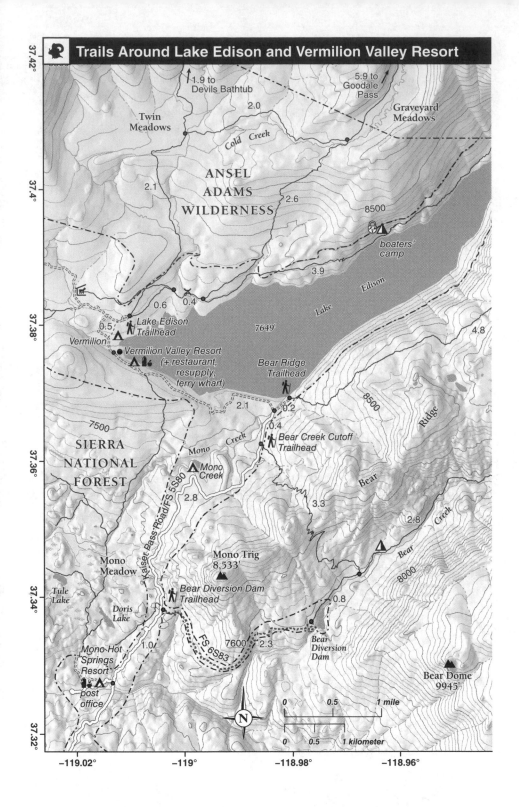

37.42°

1.9 to
Devils Bathtub

5.9 to
Goodale
Pass

2.0

Graveyard
Meadows

Twin
Meadows

Cold Creek

ANSEL
ADAMS
WILDERNESS

2.1

2.6

8500

boaters'
camp

3.9

37.4°

Lake Edison

0.6   0.4

0.5

Lake Edison
Trailhead

4.8

Vermilion

7649'

Vermilion Valley Resort
(+ restaurant,
resupply,
ferry wharf)

Bear Ridge
Trailhead

37.38°

8500

2.1   0.2

Ridge

7500

Mono   Creek

0.4

Bear Creek Cutoff
Trailhead

SIERRA
NATIONAL
FOREST

Mono
Creek

Bear

Kaiser Pass Road/FS 5S80

2.8

3.3

2.8

Bear   Creek

37.36°

Mono Trig
8,533'

8000

Mono
Meadow

Bear Diversion Dam
Trailhead

0.8

37.34°

Tule
Lake

Doris
Lake

FS 6S83

7600   2.3

Bear
Diversion
Dam

Mono Hot
Springs
Resort

1.0

Bear Dome
9945'

post
office

N

0   0.5   1 mile

0   0.5   1 kilometer

37.32°

−119.02°   −119°   −118.98°   −118.96°

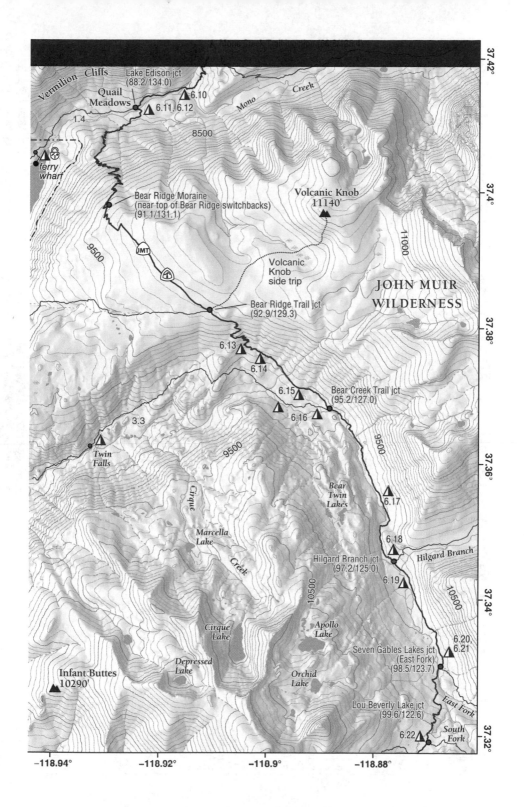

Vermilion Cliffs

Lake Edison jct
(88.2/134.0)

△ 6.10

Quail
Meadows

△ 6.11, 6.12

1.4

Mono   Creek

8500

ferry
wharf

Bear Ridge Moraine
(near top of Bear Ridge switchbacks)
(91.1/131.1)

Volcanic Knob
11140'

9500

JMT

Volcanic
Knob
side trip

JOHN MUIR
WILDERNESS

Bear Ridge Trail jct
(92.9/129.3)

11000

6.13 △

△ 6.14

6.15 △

Bear Creek Trail jct
(95.2/127.0)

△ 6.16

3.3

Twin
Falls

9500

9500

Cirque

Bear
Twin
Lakes

△ 6.17

Marcella
Lake

6.18 △

Creek

Hilgard Branch

Hilgard Branch jct
(97.2/125.0)

6.19 △

Cirque
Lake

10500

Apollo
Lake

10500

Infant Buttes
10290'

Depressed
Lake

Orchid
Lake

Seven Gables Lakes jct
(East Fork)
(98.5/123.7)

6.20,
△ 6.21

East Fork

Lou Beverly Lake jct
(99.6/122.6)

6.22 △

South
Fork

37.42°
37.4°
37.38°
37.36°
37.34°
37.32°

−118.94°   −118.92°   −118.9°   −118.88°

Trail	Trail Length (Miles)	Elevation Gain/ Loss (Feet)	Trailhead Name/ GPS Coordinates	Trailhead Elevation (Feet)	JMT Junction	N–S Distance (Miles)	S–N Distance (Miles)	Permits	Towns Accessed
Sunrise Lakes	5.2	+660/-1,820	Sunrise Lakes Trailhead (37.82574°N, 119.47004°W)	8,170	Sunrise Lakes junction	13.0	209.2	Yosemite NP: Sunrise Lakes	Tuolumne Meadows
Cathedral Lakes	0.1	+0/-20	Cathedral Lakes Trailhead (37.87337°N, 119.38251°W)	8,560	trail to Cathedral Lakes trailhead	20.5	201.7	Yosemite NP: Cathedral Lakes	Tuolumne Meadows
Lyell Canyon*	0.0	+0/-5	Tuolumne Meadows Wilderness Center (37.87658°N, 119.34569°W)	8,645	Tuolumne Meadows permit station	23.6	198.6	Yosemite NP: Lyell Canyon	Tuolumne Meadows
Rush Creek	9.2	+770/-3,170	Rush Creek Trailhead (37.78332°N, 119.12813°W)	7,240	Rush Creek junction	39.9	182.3	Inyo NF: Rush Creek	June Lake
Rush Creek	7.3	+780/-3,380	Rush Creek Trailhead (37.78332°N, 119.12813°W)	7,240	Thousand Island Lake junction	43.1	179.1	Inyo NF: Rush Creek	June Lake
High Trail to Agnew Meadows	8.2	+850/-2,340	High Trailhead (37.68282°N, 119.08471°W)	8,330	Thousand Island Lake junction	43.1	179.1	Inyo NF: High Trail	Mammoth Lakes
River Trail to Agnew Meadows	7.5	+560/-2,090	River Trailhead (37.68184°N, 119.08621°W);	8,310	Thousand Island Lake junction	43.1	179.1	Inyo NF: River Trail	Mammoth Lakes
Shadow Creek to Agnew Meadows	4.1	+440/-900	River Trailhead (37.68184°N, 119.08621°W)	8,310	Shadow Lake junction	49.2	173	Inyo NF: Shadow Creek	Mammoth Lakes
Devils Postpile	0.75 (N), 0.6 (S)	+135/-25 (N), +160/-25 (S)	Devils Postpile Ranger Station (37.62978°N, 119.08465°W)	7,560	northern (or southern) Devils Postpile junction	59.4 (57.8)	165.1 (164.4)	Inyo NF: JMT South of Devils Postpile if southbound; JMT North of Devils Postpile northbound	northbound Mammoth Lakes, Devils Postpile
Reds Meadow Resort to JMT*	0.3 (W), 0.35 (E)	+80/-0	Reds Meadow Resort (37.61296°N, 119.02134°W)	7,700	western (or eastern) Reds Meadow junction	59.4 (59.5)	162.8 (162.7)	Inyo NF: JMT South of Devils Postpile if southbound; JMT North of Devils Postpile northbound	northbound Mammoth Lakes, Reds Meadow Resort
Mammoth Pass from Lower Crater Meadow	3.3	+780/-410	Horseshoe Lake (37.61296°N, 119.02134°W)	9,010	lower Crater Meadow junction (Mammoth Pass)	62.2	160.0	Inyo NF: Red Cones	Mammoth Lakes

*Common resupply point

North-to-south distances are in miles from Happy Isles, while south-to-north distances are in miles from Whitney Portal.

Abbreviations: NP = National Park • NF = National Forest • SEKI = Sequoia and Kings Canyon National Parks

Trail	Trail Length (Miles)	Elevation Gain/Loss (Feet)	Trailhead Name/GPS Coordinates	Trailhead Elevation (Feet)	JMT Junction	N–S Distance (Miles)	S–N Distance (Miles)	Permits	Towns/Lodging Accessed
Mammoth Pass from Upper Crater Meadow	3.6	+770/-670	Horseshoe Lake (37.61296°N, 119.02134°W)	9,010	Upper Crater Meadow junction (Mammoth Pass)	62.9	159.3	Inyo NF: Red Cones	Mammoth Lakes
Duck Pass	5.7	+790/-1,810	Coldwater Campground Duck Pass Trailhead (37.59122°N, 118.98925°W)	9,140	Duck Pass junction	70.6	151.6	Inyo NF: Duck Pass	Mammoth Lakes
McGee Pass	15.1	+3,050/-4,700	McGee Pass Trailhead (37.55102°N, 118.80254°W)	7,870	McGee Pass junction (Tully Hole)	76.9	145.3	Inyo NF: McGee Pass	Mammoth Lakes
Fish Creek Trail and Iva Bell Hot Springs	18.4	+3,220/-4,730	Reds Meadow Resort (37.61296°N, 119.02134°W)	7,700	Cascade Valley (Fish Creek) junction	78.0	144.2	Inyo NF: Fish Creek	Mammoth Lakes, Reds Meadow Resort
Goodale Pass	11.1	+830/-3,580	Lake Edison (Mono Creek) Trailhead (37.38122°N, 119.01035°W)	7,800	Goodale Pass junction	80.7	141.5	Sierra NF: Mono Creek Trail	Lake Edison, Vermilion Valley Resort (VVR)
Mono Pass	15.9	+4,380/-2,480	Mono Pass Trailhead (Mosquito Flat) (37.435519°N, 118.74720°W)	10,240	Mono Creek junction	86.8	135.4	Inyo NF: Mono Pass	Mammoth Lakes, Bishop
Lake Edison*	1.5 (to ferry) 6.3 (to TH)	+900/-990 (TH)	Lake Edison (Mono Creek) Trailhead (37.38122°N, 119.01035°W)	7,800	Lake Edison (Quail Meadows) junction	88.2	134.0	Sierra NF: Mono Creek Trail	Lake Thomas Edison, VVR
Bear Ridge	4.8	+120/-2,330	Bear Ridge Trailhead (near Lake Edison dam) (37.36906°N, 118.98052°W)	7,660	Bear Ridge junction	92.9	129.3	Sierra NF: Bear Ridge	Lake Thomas Edison, VVR
Bear Creek to Bear Cutoff	9.2	+1,190/-2,580	Bear Cutoff Trailhead (Lake Edison Road fairly near dam) (37.36255°N, 118.98589°W)	7,560	Bear Creek junction	95.2	127.0	Sierra NF: Bear Diversion	Lake Thomas Edison, VVR

Trail	Trail Length (Miles)	Elevation Gain/ Loss (Feet)	Trailhead Name/ GPS Coordinates	Trailhead Elevation (Feet)	JMT Junction	N–S Distance (Miles)	S–N Distance (Miles)	Permits	Towns Accessed
Bear Creek to Diversion Dam	9.5	+610/–2,530	Bear Diversion Trailhead (Lake Edison Road near Mono Meadows) (37.33823°N, 119.00438°W)	7,010	Bear Creek junction	95.2	127.0	Sierra NF: Bear Diversion	Lake Thomas Edison, Mono Hot Springs, VVR
Hilgard Branch and Italy Pass	17.8	+3,920/–5,800	Pine Creek Trailhead (37.36101°N, 118.6922°W)	7,440	Hilgard Branch junction	97.2	125.0	Inyo NF: Italy Pass	Bishop
Florence Lake*	6.2 (to ferry) 10.1 (to TH)	+450/–990 (to ferry); +1,130/–1,670 (to TH)	Florence Lake ferry wharf (37.25040°N, 118.94129°W), Florence Lake Trailhead (37.27665°N, 118.97636°W)	7,330' (ferry), 7,350' (TH)	southern (or northern) Muir Trail Ranch cutoff	108.5 (N) 110.3 (S)	113.7 (N) 111.9 (S)	Sierra NF: Florence	Florence Lake, Muir Trail Ranch
Pine Creek Pass	17.8	+3,810/–4,450	Pine Creek Trailhead (37.36101°N, 118.6922°W)	7,440	Piute Creek junction	112.1	110.1	Inyo NF: Pine Creek	Bishop
Piute Pass	16.9	+3,940/–2,670	Piute Pass Trailhead (North Lake) (37.227731°N, 118.62746°W)	9,360	Piute Creek junction	112.1	110.1	Inyo NF: Piute Pass	Bishop
Lamarck Col	9.2	+2,630/–3,900	Piute Pass Trailhead (North Lake) (37.227731°N, 118.62746°W)	9,360	Piute Creek junction	123.2	99.0	Inyo NF: Piute Pass	Bishop
Bishop Pass	12.3	+3,520/–2,450	Bishop Pass Trailhead (South Lake) (37.16934°N, 118.56580°W)	9,820	Bishop Pass junction	137.8	84.4	Inyo NF: Bishop Pass - South Lake	Bishop
Taboose Pass	10.0	+820/–6,160	Taboose Pass Trailhead (37.00957°N, 118.32736°W)	5,420	Taboose Pass junction	158.9	63.3	Inyo NF: Taboose Pass	Big Pine, Independence
Sawmill Pass	13.1	+1,410/–7,180	Sawmill Pass Trailhead (36.93891°N, 118.29029°W)	4,600	Sawmill Pass junction	165.9	56.3	Inyo NF: Sawmill Pass	Big Pine, Independence

*Common resupply point

Trail	Trail Length (Miles)	Elevation Gain/ Loss (Feet)	Trailhead Name/ GPS Coordinates	Trailhead Elevation (Feet)	JMT Junction	N–S Distance (Miles)	S–N Distance (Miles)	Permits	Towns Accessed
Woods Creek	14.5	−760/−4,280	Roads End, Cedar Grove (36.79461°N, 118.58299°W)	5,020	Woods Creek junction	169.6	52.6	SEKI: Woods Creek	Cedar Grove (Kings Canyon NP)
Baxter Pass	11.9	+2,430/−6,600	Baxter Pass Trailhead (36.84478°N, 118.29765°W)	6,040	Baxter Pass junction	173.6	48.6	Inyo NF: Baxter Pass	Independence
Kearsarge Pass (from N)*	7.7	+1,270/−2,840	Kearsarge Pass Trailhead (Onion Valley) (36.77254°N, 118.34107°W)	9,200	Kearsarge Pass (or Charlotte Lake) junction	180.6	41.6	Inyo NF: Kearsarge Pass	Independence
Kearsarge Pass (via Kearsarge Lakes)*	7.5	+1,480/−2,800	Kearsarge Pass Trailhead (Onion Valley) (36.77254°N, 118.34107°W)	9,200	Bullfrog Lake junction	181.2	41.0	Inyo NF: Kearsarge Pass	Independence
Bubbs Creek	12.6	+330/−4,880	Roads End, Cedar Grove (36.79461°N, 118.58299°W)	5,020	Bubbs Creek junction (Lower Vidette Meadow)	182.4	39.8	SEKI: Bubbs Creek	Cedar Grove (Kings Canyon NP)
Shepherd Pass	13.9	+1,870/−6,480	Shepherd Pass Trailhead 36.72708°N, 118.27888°W	6,313'	Shepherd Pass junction	195.5	26.7	Inyo NF: Shepherd Pass	Independence
New Army Pass, Cottonwood Lakes**	22.6	+4,040/−4,750	Cottonwood Lakes Trailhead (in Horseshoe Meadows, 36.45321°N, 118.17005°W)	10,060'	PCT junction west of Crabtree Meadow	203.3	18.9	Inyo NF: Cottonwood Lakes	Lone Pine
Cottonwood Pass**	20.5	+3,360/−4,190	Cottonwood Pass Trailhead (in Horseshoe Meadows, 36.44834°N, 118.17070°W)	9,950'	PCT junction west of Crabtree Meadow	203.3	18.9	Inyo NF: Cottonwood Pass	Lone Pine

**Alternative starting point

Tenaya Lake, from Sunrise Lakes High Sierra Camp

LEAVE JMT AT: 13.0/209.2

ACCESS TO: Tenaya Lake at Sunrise Lakes Trailhead (37.82574°N, 119.47004°W)

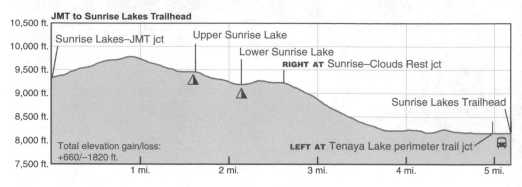

Tuolumne Meadows, from Cathedral Lakes

LEAVE JMT AT: 20.5/201.7

ACCESS TO: Tuolumne Meadows at Cathedral Lakes Trailhead (37.87337°N, 119.38251°W). See map on page 11.

Tuolumne Meadows, from Lyell Canyon

LEAVE JMT AT: 23.6/198.6

ACCESS TO: Tuolumne Meadows at Wilderness Center parking area (37.87658°N, 119.34569°W). See map on page 11.

Rush Creek Trailhead via Waugh Lake

LEAVE JMT AT: 39.9/182.3

ACCESS TO: Rush Creek Trailhead near June Lake (37.78332°N, 119.12813°W)

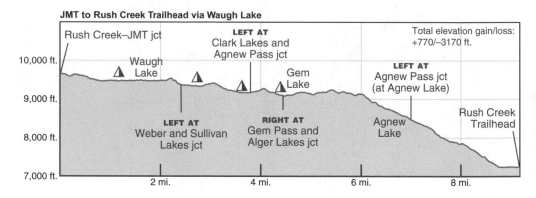

Rush Creek Trailhead from Thousand Island Lake

LEAVE JMT AT: 43.1/179.1

ACCESS TO: Rush Creek Trailhead near June Lake (37.78332°N, 119.12813°W). See elevation profile at the top of the next page.

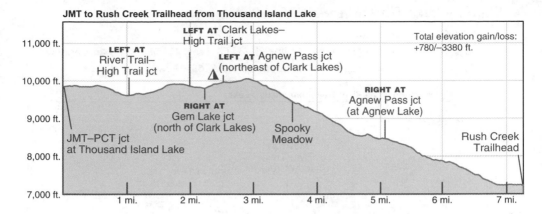

Agnew Meadows (via High Trail) from Thousand Island Lake

LEAVE JMT AT: 43.1/179.1

ACCESS TO: Agnew Meadows (High Trailhead) (37.68282°N, 119.08471°W) and Agnew Meadows shuttle bus stop (near Mammoth Lakes) (37.68109°N, 119.08082°W)

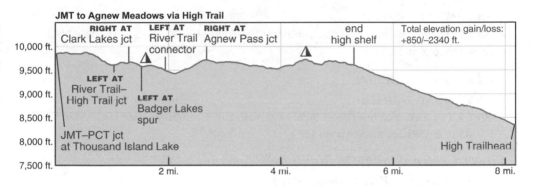

Agnew Meadows (via River Trail) from Thousand Island Lake

LEAVE JMT AT: 43.1/179.1

ACCESS TO: Agnew Meadows (River Trailhead) (37.68184°N, 119.08621°W) and Agnew Meadows shuttle bus stop (near Mammoth Lakes) (37.68109°N, 119.08082°W)

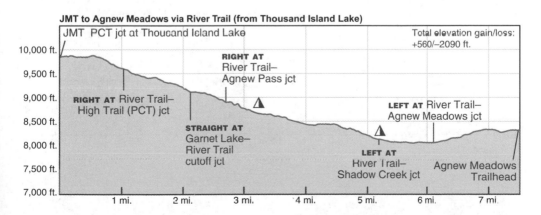

Shadow Lake Trail to Agnew Meadows

LEAVE JMT AT: 49.2/173.0

ACCESS TO: Agnew Meadows (River Trailhead) (37.68184°N, 119.08621°W) and Agnew Meadows shuttle bus stop (near Mammoth Lakes) (37.68109°N, 119.08082°W)

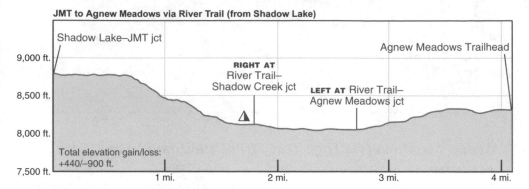

Devils Postpile

LEAVE JMT AT: 57.1/164.4

ACCESS TO: Devils Postpile Ranger Station (near Mammoth Lakes) (37.62978°N, 119.08465°W). See map on page 13.

Red's Meadow Resort

LEAVE JMT AT: 59.4/162.8

ACCESS TO: Red's Meadow Resort (near Mammoth Lakes, resupply pickup) (37.61476°N, 119.07508°W). See map on page 13.

Lower Crater Meadow to Mammoth Pass and on to Horseshoe Lake (Red Cones Trailhead)

LEAVE JMT AT: 62.2/160.0

ACCESS TO: Horseshoe Lake in Mammoth Lakes Basin (37.61296°N, 119.02134°W)

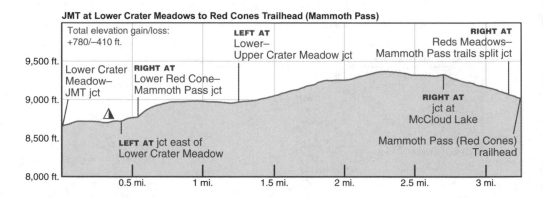

Upper Crater Meadow to Mammoth Pass and on to Horseshoe Lake (Red Cones Trailhead)

LEAVE JMT AT: 62.9/159.3

ACCESS TO: Horseshoe Lake in Mammoth Lakes Basin (37.61296°N, 119.02134°W)

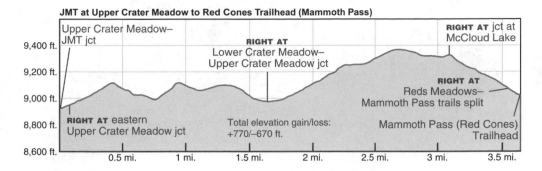

Duck Pass Trail

LEAVE JMT AT: 70.6/151.6

ACCESS TO: Mammoth Lakes Basin; Coldwater Campground/Duck Pass Trailhead (37.59122°N, 118.98925°W)

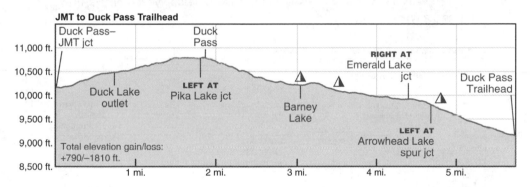

McGee Pass Trail

LEAVE JMT AT: 76.9/145.3

ACCESS TO: Crowley Lake region, 8 miles south of Mammoth Lakes on US 395; McGee Pass Trailhead (37.55102°N, 118.80254°W). See elevation profile at the top of the next page.

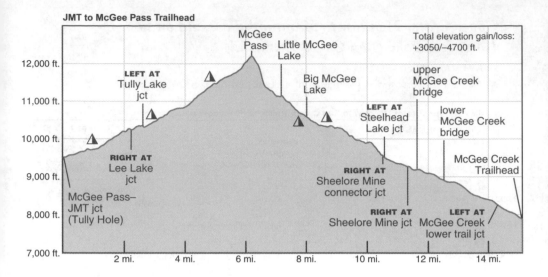

JMT to McGee Pass Trailhead

Labels in elevation profile (top to bottom, left to right):

McGee Pass
Little McGee Lake

Total elevation gain/loss: +3050/–4700 ft.

LEFT AT Tully Lake jct

Big McGee Lake

upper McGee Creek bridge

LEFT AT Steelhead Lake jct

lower McGee Creek bridge

RIGHT AT Lee Lake jct

McGee Creek Trailhead

McGee Pass– JMT jct (Tully Hole)

RIGHT AT Sheelore Mine connector jct

RIGHT AT Sheelore Mine jct

LEFT AT McGee Creek lower trail jct

Fish Creek Trail to Cascade Valley, Iva Bell Hot Springs, and Ultimately Reds Meadow

LEAVE JMT AT: 78.0/144.2

ACCESS TO: Red's Meadow Resort near Mammoth Lakes (resupply pickup) (37.61476°N, 119.07508°W)

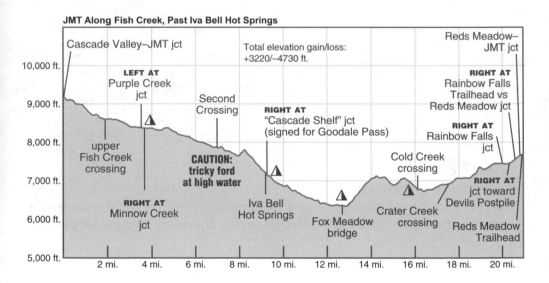

JMT Along Fish Creek, Past Iva Bell Hot Springs

Labels in elevation profile:

Cascade Valley–JMT jct

Reds Meadow– JMT jct

Total elevation gain/loss: +3220/–4730 ft.

LEFT AT Purple Creek jct

RIGHT AT Rainbow Falls Trailhead vs Reds Meadow jct

Second Crossing

RIGHT AT "Cascade Shelf" jct (signed for Goodale Pass)

RIGHT AT Rainbow Falls jct

upper Fish Creek crossing

CAUTION: tricky ford at high water

Cold Creek crossing

RIGHT AT jct toward Devils Postpile

RIGHT AT Minnow Creek jct

Iva Bell Hot Springs

Fox Meadow bridge

Crater Creek crossing

Reds Meadow Trailhead

Goodale Pass

LEAVE JMT AT: 80.7/141.5

ACCESS TO: Lake Edison, Vermilion Valley Resort (resupply pickup) (37.37625°N, 119.01250°W); Lake Edison Trailhead (37.38122°N, 119.01035°W). See elevation profile at the top of the next page.

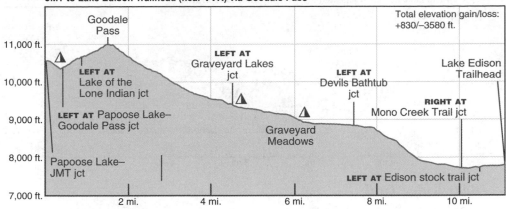

JMT to Lake Edison Trailhead (near VVR) via Goodale Pass

Total elevation gain/loss: +830/−3580 ft.

Goodale Pass

LEFT AT Lake of the Lone Indian jct

LEFT AT Graveyard Lakes jct

LEFT AT Devils Bathtub jct

Lake Edison Trailhead

RIGHT AT Mono Creek Trail jct

LEFT AT Papoose Lake–Goodale Pass jct

Graveyard Meadows

Papoose Lake–JMT jct

LEFT AT Edison stock trail jct

Mono Pass Trail

LEAVE JMT AT: 86.8/135.4

ACCESS TO: Mosquito Flat Trailhead (37.43519°N, 118.74720°W) and beyond to Toms Place, 24 miles north of Bishop and 15 miles south of Mammoth Lakes on US 395

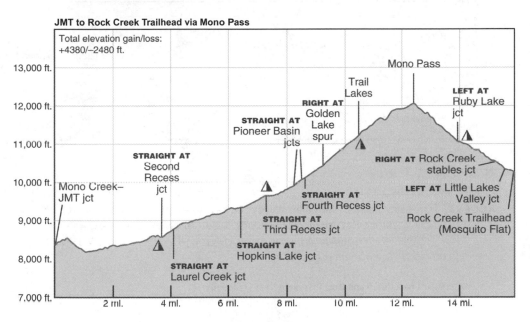

JMT to Rock Creek Trailhead via Mono Pass

Total elevation gain/loss: +4380/−2480 ft.

Mono Pass

Trail Lakes

RIGHT AT Golden Lake spur

STRAIGHT AT Pioneer Basin jcts

LEFT AT Ruby Lake jct

STRAIGHT AT Second Recess jct

RIGHT AT Rock Creek stables jct

Mono Creek–JMT jct

STRAIGHT AT Fourth Recess jct

LEFT AT Little Lakes Valley jct

STRAIGHT AT Third Recess jct

Rock Creek Trailhead (Mosquito Flat)

STRAIGHT AT Hopkins Lake jct

STRAIGHT AT Laurel Creek jct

Lake Edison Trail

LEAVE JMT AT: 88.2/134.0

ACCESS TO: Lake Edison, Vermilion Valley Resort (resupply pickup) (37.37625°N, 119.01250°W); Lake Edison Trailhead (37.38122°N, 119.01035°W). See elevation profile at the top of the next page and map on pages 82–83.

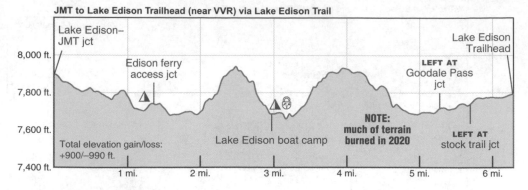

Bear Ridge Trail

LEAVE JMT AT: 92.9/129.3

ACCESS TO: Lake Edison, Vermilion Valley Resort (resupply pickup) (37.37625°N, 119.01250°W), Mono Hot Springs (37.32703°N, 119.01761°W); Bear Ridge Trailhead near Vermilion Valley (Lake Edison) Dam (37.36906°N, 118.98052°W). See map on pages 82–83.

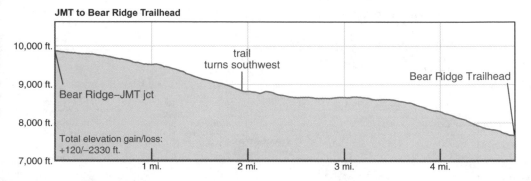

Bear Creek Trail

LEAVE JMT AT: 95.2/127.0

ACCESS TO: Lake Edison, Vermilion Valley Resort (resupply pickup) (37.37625°N, 119.01250°W); Mono Hot Springs (37.32703°N, 119.01761°W); Bear Creek Cutoff Trailhead (37.36255°N, 118.98589°W); Bear Creek Diversion Dam Trailhead (37.33823°N, 119.00438°W). See map on pages 82–83.

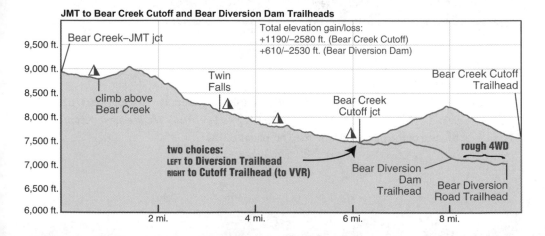

Hilgard Branch to Italy Pass (Use Trail) and Pine Creek Trailhead

LEAVE JMT AT: 97.2/125.0

ACCESS TO: US 395, 10 miles north of Bishop; Pine Creek Trailhead (37.36101°N, 118.6922°W).
See map on pages 32–33.

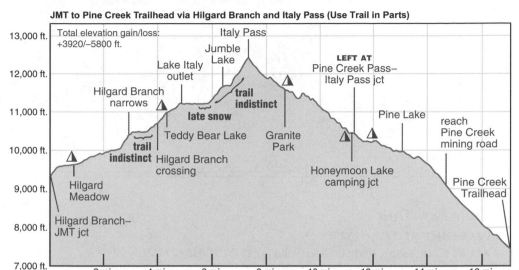

JMT to Pine Creek Trailhead via Hilgard Branch and Italy Pass (Use Trail in Parts)

Florence Lake Trail Past Muir Trail Ranch

LEAVE JMT AT: 108.5/110.3

ACCESS TO: Muir Trail Ranch (resupply pickup) (37.23611°N, 118.88115°W); Florence Lake ferry
wharf (37.25040°N, 118.94129°W); Florence Lake Trailhead (37.27665°N, 118.97636°W)

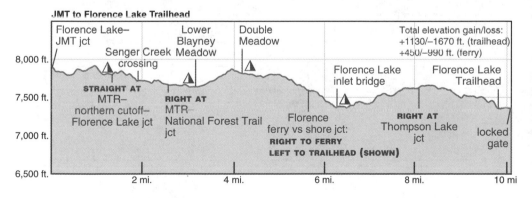

JMT to Florence Lake Trailhead

Pine Creek Pass Trail

LEAVE JMT AT: 112.1/110.1

ACCESS TO: US 395, 10 miles north of Bishop; Pine Creek Trailhead (37.36101°N, 118.6922°W).
See elevation profile at the top of the next page.

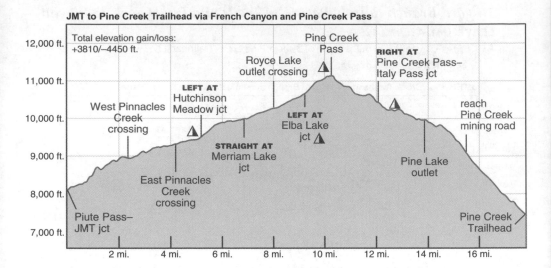

JMT to Pine Creek Trailhead via French Canyon and Pine Creek Pass

Total elevation gain/loss: +3810/–4450 ft.

Piute Pass Trail

LEAVE JMT AT: 112.1/110.1

ACCESS TO: Bishop; North Lake Trailhead (37.22731°N, 118.62746°W)

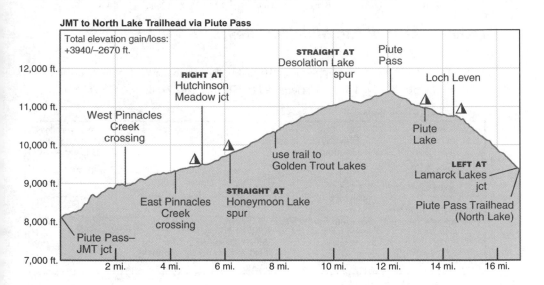

JMT to North Lake Trailhead via Piute Pass

Total elevation gain/loss: +3940/–2670 ft.

Lamarck Col

LEAVE JMT AT: 123.2/99.0

ACCESS TO: Bishop; North Lake Trailhead (37.22731°N, 118.62746°W). See elevation profile at the top of the next page and map on pages 36–37.

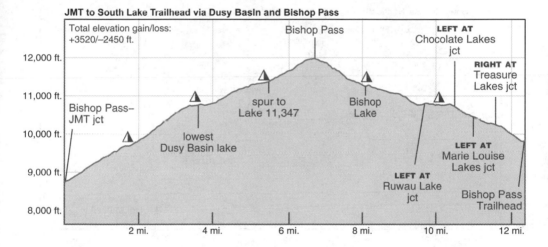

JMT to North Lake Trailhead via Lamarck Col (**NOTE:** rough use trail; difficult route)

Total elevation gain/loss: +2630/−3900 ft.

- Lamarck Col
- Darwin Bench
- persistent snowbank
- cross ridge into Upper Lamarck Lake drainage
- boulders
- Lower Lamarck Lake
- Darwin Canyon Lake 11,592
- LEFT AT Grass Lake jct
- CAUTION: use trail from JMT to Upper Lamarck Lake; unmarked and in places inobvious
- RIGHT AT Upper Lamarck Lake spur
- Lamarck Col–JMT jct
- RIGHT AT Piute Pass jct
- Piute Pass Trailhead

13,000 ft. / 12,000 ft. / 11,000 ft. / 10,000 ft. / 9,000 ft. / 8,000 ft.

2 mi. / 4 mi. / 6 mi. / 8 mi.

Bishop Pass Trail

LEAVE JMT AT: 137.8/84.4

ACCESS TO: Bishop; South Lake Trailhead (37.16934°N, 118.56580°W)

JMT to South Lake Trailhead via Dusy Basin and Bishop Pass

Total elevation gain/loss: +3520/−2450 ft.

- Bishop Pass
- LEFT AT Chocolate Lakes jct
- RIGHT AT Treasure Lakes jct
- Bishop Pass–JMT jct
- spur to Lake 11,347
- Bishop Lake
- lowest Dusy Basin lake
- LEFT AT Marie Louise Lakes jct
- LEFT AT Ruwau Lake jct
- Bishop Pass Trailhead

12,000 ft. / 11,000 ft. / 10,000 ft. / 9,000 ft. / 8,000 ft.

2 mi. / 4 mi. / 6 mi. / 8 mi. / 10 mi. / 12 mi.

Taboose Pass Trail

LEAVE JMT AT: 158.9/63.3

ACCESS TO: US 395, 12 miles south of Big Pine, 14 miles north of Independence; Taboose Pass Trailhead (37.00957°N, 118.32736°W) . See elevation profile at the top of the next page.

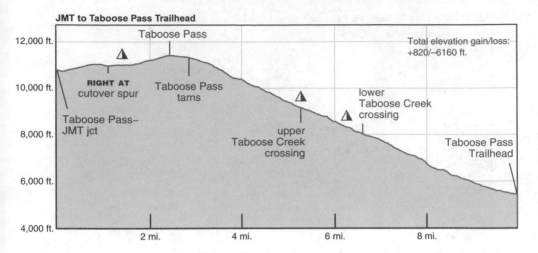

JMT to Taboose Pass Trailhead

Taboose Pass

Total elevation gain/loss:
+820/−6160 ft.

12,000 ft.

10,000 ft. — **RIGHT AT** cutover spur — Taboose Pass tarns — lower Taboose Creek crossing

Taboose Pass–JMT jct

8,000 ft. — upper Taboose Creek crossing — Taboose Pass Trailhead

6,000 ft.

4,000 ft.

2 mi.   4 mi.   6 mi.   8 mi.

Sawmill Pass Trail

LEAVE JMT AT: 165.9/56.3

ACCESS TO: US 395, 18.0 miles south of Big Pine, 8.5 miles north of Independence;
Sawmill Pass Trailhead (36.93891°N, 118.29029°W)

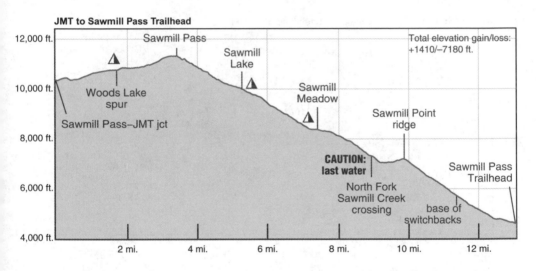

JMT to Sawmill Pass Trailhead

Sawmill Pass

Sawmill Lake

Total elevation gain/loss:
+1410/−7180 ft.

12,000 ft.

10,000 ft. — Woods Lake spur — Sawmill Meadow

Sawmill Pass–JMT jct

Sawmill Point ridge

8,000 ft.

CAUTION: last water

Sawmill Pass Trailhead

6,000 ft. — North Fork Sawmill Creek crossing — base of switchbacks

4,000 ft.

2 mi.   4 mi.   6 mi.   8 mi.   10 mi.   12 mi.

Woods Creek Trail

LEAVE JMT AT: 169.6/52.6

ACCESS TO: Roads End at Cedar Grove in Kings Canyon National Park (36.79461°N,
118.58290°W). See elevation profile at the top of the next page.

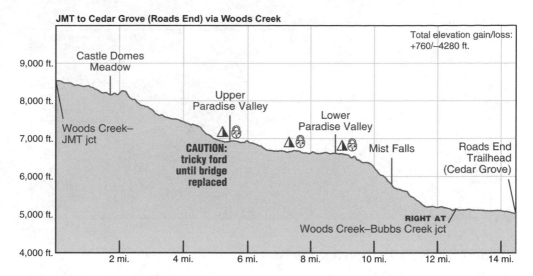

JMT to Cedar Grove (Roads End) via Woods Creek

Total elevation gain/loss: +760/–4280 ft.

Castle Domes Meadow

Upper Paradise Valley

Lower Paradise Valley

Woods Creek–JMT jct

CAUTION: tricky ford until bridge replaced

Mist Falls

Roads End Trailhead (Cedar Grove)

RIGHT AT
Woods Creek–Bubbs Creek jct

Baxter Pass Trail

LEAVE JMT AT: 173.6/48.6

ACCESS TO: Independence; Baxter Pass Trailhead (36.84478°N, 118.29765°W)

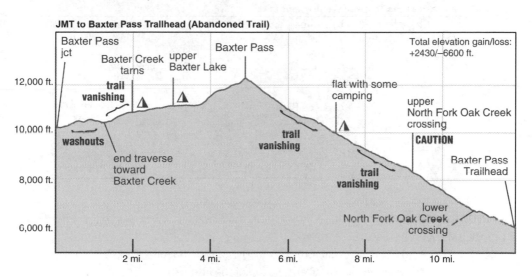

JMT to Baxter Pass Trailhead (Abandoned Trail)

Baxter Pass jct

Baxter Creek tarns

upper Baxter Lake

Baxter Pass

Total elevation gain/loss: +2430/–6600 ft.

trail vanishing

flat with some camping

upper North Fork Oak Creek crossing

washouts

end traverse toward Baxter Creek

trail vanishing

CAUTION

Baxter Pass Trailhead

trail vanishing

lower North Fork Oak Creek crossing

Kearsarge Pass Trail, from the North

LEAVE JMT AT: 180.6/41.6

ACCESS TO: Onion Valley near Independence; Kearsarge Pass Trailhead (36.77254°N, 118.34107°W). See elevation profile at the top of the next page.

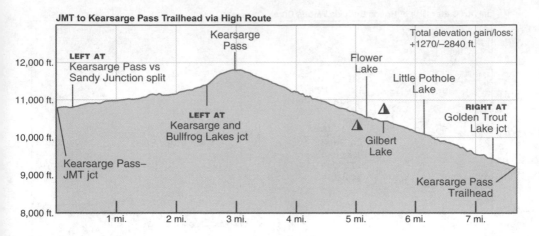

JMT to Kearsarge Pass Trailhead via High Route

Kearsarge Pass Trail, from the South

LEAVE JMT AT: 181.2/41.0

ACCESS TO: Onion Valley near Independence; Kearsarge Pass Trailhead (36.77254°N, 118.34107°W)

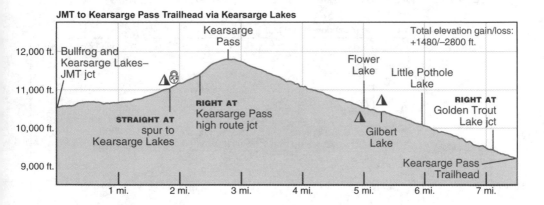

JMT to Kearsarge Pass Trailhead via Kearsarge Lakes

Bubbs Creek Trail

LEAVE JMT AT: 182.4/39.8

ACCESS TO: Roads End at Cedar Grove in Kings Canyon National Park (36.79461°N, 118.58290°W). See elevation profile at the top of the next page.

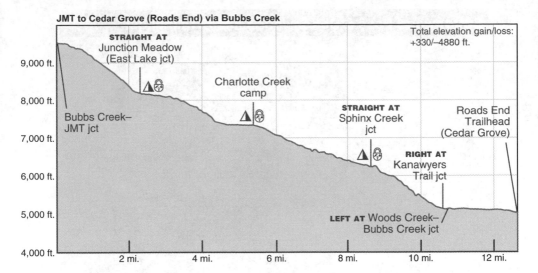

JMT to Cedar Grove (Roads End) via Bubbs Creek

Total elevation gain/loss: +330/−4880 ft.

STRAIGHT AT Junction Meadow (East Lake jct)

Charlotte Creek camp

STRAIGHT AT Sphinx Creek jct

Roads End Trailhead (Cedar Grove)

Bubbs Creek– JMT jct

RIGHT AT Kanawyers Trail jct

LEFT AT Woods Creek– Bubbs Creek jct

Shepherd Pass Trail

LEAVE JMT AT: 195.5/26.7

ACCESS TO: Shepherd Pass Trailhead near Independence (36.72708°N, 118.27888°W)

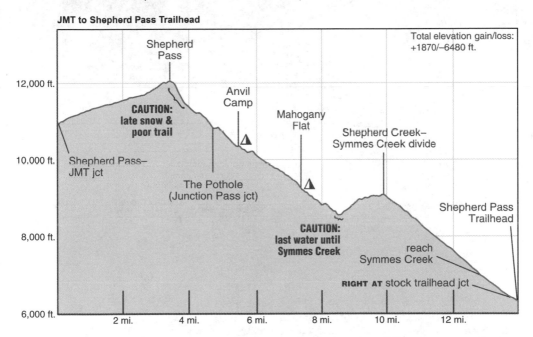

JMT to Shepherd Pass Trailhead

Total elevation gain/loss: +1870/−6480 ft.

Shepherd Pass

Anvil Camp

CAUTION: late snow & poor trail

Mahogany Flat

Shepherd Creek– Symmes Creek divide

Shepherd Pass– JMT jct

The Pothole (Junction Pass jct)

Shepherd Pass Trailhead

CAUTION: last water until Symmes Creek

reach Symmes Creek

RIGHT AT stock trailhead jct

PCT South, from Crabtree to Cottonwood Lakes

LEAVE JMT AT: 203.3/18.9

ACCESS TO: Lone Pine; Cottonwood Lakes Trailhead in Horseshoe Meadows (36.45321°N, 118.17006°W). This is a popular alternative way to begin (or end) a JMT hike if you cannot get a permit for Whitney Portal. See maps on the next four pages and elevation profile at the top of page 106. *(continued on page 106)*

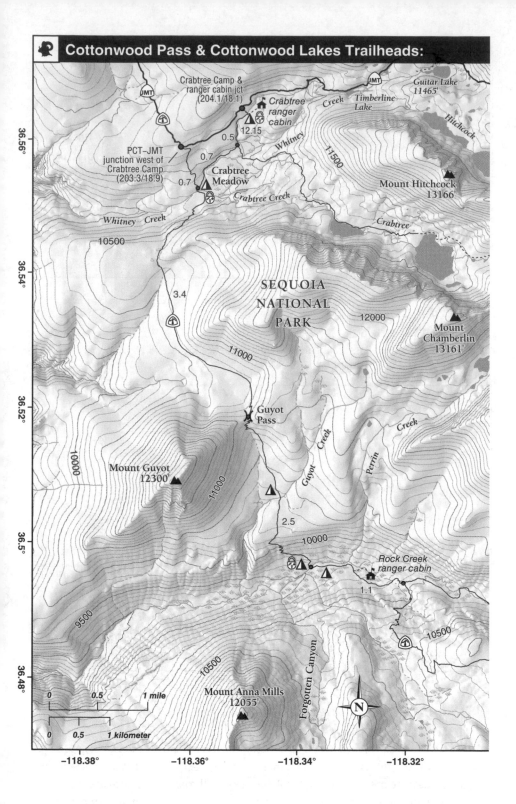

JMT

Crabtree Camp &
ranger cabin jct
(204.1/18.1)

Crabtree
ranger
cabin

12.15

JMT

Guitar Lake
11465'

Creek

Timberline
Lake

Hitchcock

Whitney

0.5

11500

0.7

PCT–JMT
junction west of
Crabtree Camp
(203.3/18.9)

0.7

Crabtree
Meadow

Mount Hitchcock
13166'

Crabtree Creek

Crabtree

Whitney   Creek

10500

SEQUOIA
NATIONAL
PARK

12000

Mount
Chamberlin
13161'

3.4

11000

Guyot
Pass

Creek

Mount Guyot
12300'

Guyot Creek

Perrin   Creek

10000

11000

2.5

10000

Rock Creek
ranger cabin

1.1

9500

10500

10500

Mount Anna Mills
12055'

Forgotten Canyon

N

0   0.5   1 mile

0   0.5   1 kilometer

−118.38°   −118.36°   −118.34°   −118.32°

36.56°

36.54°

36.52°

36.5°

36.48°

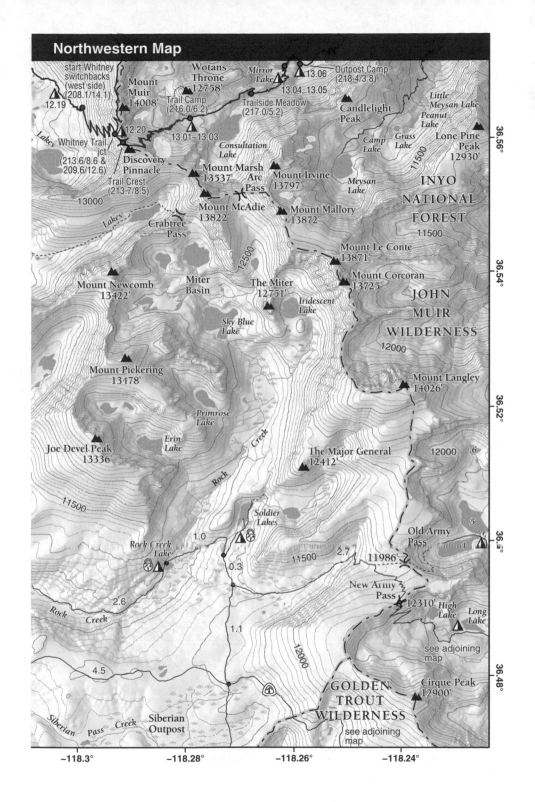

start Whitney
switchbacks
(west side)
(208.1/14.1)
12.19

Mount
Muir
14008'

Wotans
Throne
12758'

Mirror
Lake

13.06

13.04, 13.05

Outpost Camp
(218.4/3.8)

Little
Meysan
Lake
Peanut
Lake

Trail Camp
(216.0/6.2)

Trailside Meadow
(217.0/5.2)

Candlelight
Peak

Lone Pine
Peak
12930'

12.20

13.01–13.03

Camp
Lake

Grass
Lake

Whitney Trail
jct
(213.6/8.6 &
209.6/12.6)

Lakes

Discovery
Pinnacle

Consultation
Lake

Mount Marsh
13537'

Arc
Pass

Mount Irvine
13797'

Meysan
Lake

INYO

NATIONAL

Trail Crest
(213.7/8.5)

13000

Mount McAdie
13822'

Mount Mallory
13872'

FOREST

11500

Lakes

Crabtree
Pass

Mount Le Conte
13871'

12500

Mount Newcomb
13422'

Miter
Basin

The Miter
12751'

Mount Corcoran
13725'

Iridescent
Lake

JOHN

MUIR

WILDERNESS

12000

Sky Blue
Lake

Mount Piekering
13178'

Primrose
Lake

Erin
Lake

Mount Langley
14026'

36.56°

36.54°

36.52°

Joe Devel Peak
13336'

11500

The Major General
12412'

12000

6

Soldier
Lakes

Old Army
Pass

5

36.5°

Rock Creek
Lake

1.0

2.7

11986'

1

0.3

11500

2.6

Rock Creek

New Army
Pass

12310'

High
Lake

Long
Lake

1.1

see adjoining
map

4.5

12000

Cirque Peak
12900'

36.48°

Siberian
Pass

Creek

Siberian
Outpost

GOLDEN
TROUT
WILDERNESS

see adjoining
map

−118.3°

−118.28°

−118.26°

−118.24°

Rock Creek

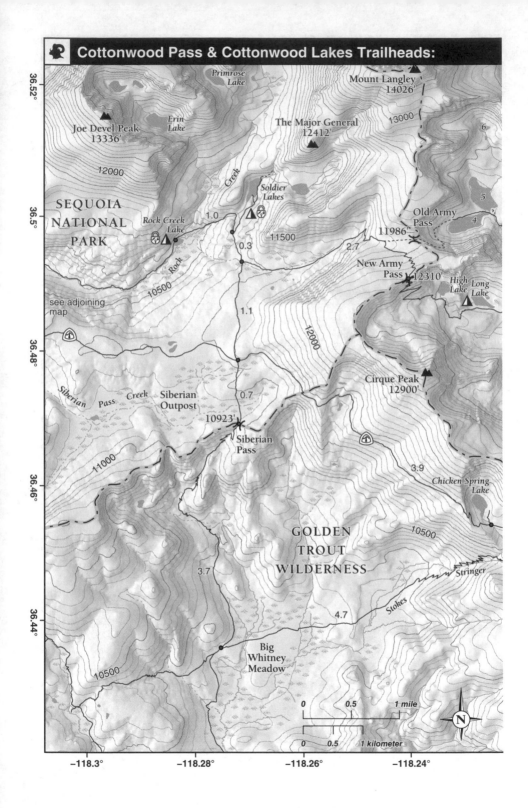

Primrose Lake

Mount Langley
14026'

Joe Devel Peak
13336'

Erin Lake

The Major General
12412'

13000

6

SEQUOIA
NATIONAL
PARK

12000

Creek

Soldier Lakes

1.0

Old Army
Pass

5

Rock Creek Lake

0.3

11500

2.7

11986'

4

New Army
Pass

12310'

High Lake

Long Lake

Rock

10500

1.1

see adjoining
map

12000

Siberian

Pass

Creek

Siberian
Outpost

0.7

Cirque Peak
12900'

10923'

Siberian
Pass

3.9

Chicken Spring
Lake

11000

GOLDEN
TROUT
WILDERNESS

10500

3.7

Stringer

4.7

Stokes

Big
Whitney
Meadow

10500

0   0.5   1 mile

N

0   0.5   1 kilometer

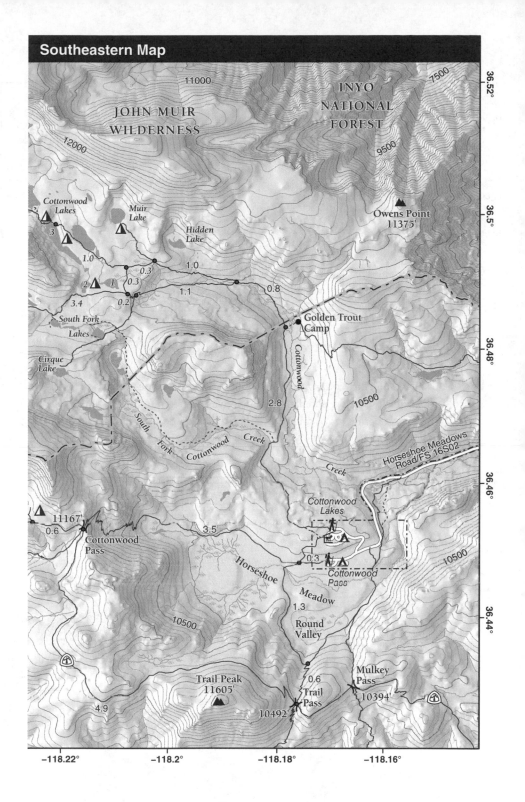

JOHN MUIR
WILDERNESS

INYO
NATIONAL
FOREST

11000

7500

12000

9500

Cottonwood
Lakes

3

Muir
Lake

Hidden
Lake

Owens Point
11375'

36.52°

36.5°

1.0

0.3

1.0

2   1

0.3

1.1

0.8

3.4

0.2

South Fork
Lakes

Golden Trout
Camp

36.48°

Cirque
Lake

2.8

10500

South Fork   Cottonwood   Creek

Horseshoe Meadows
Road/FS 16S02

Creek

36.46°

11167'

0.6

Cottonwood
Pass

3.5

Cottonwood
Lakes

10500

Horseshoe

0.3

Cottonwood
Pass

10500

Meadow

1.3

Round
Valley

Trail Peak
11605'

Mulkey
Pass

10394'

4.9

0.6

Trail
Pass

10492'

36.44°

−118.22°   −118.2°   −118.18°   −118.16°

(continued from page 101)

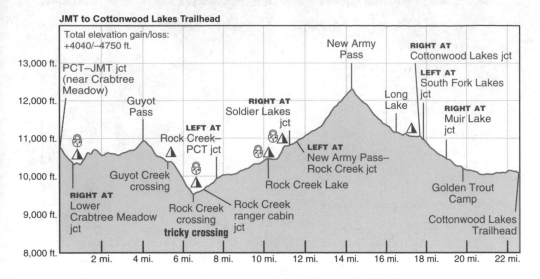

JMT to Cottonwood Lakes Trailhead

PCT South, from Crabtree to Cottonwood Pass

LEAVE JMT AT: 203.3/18.9

ACCESS TO: Lone Pine; Cottonwood Pass Trailhead in Horseshoe Meadows (36.44834°N, 118.17070°W). This is a popular alternative way to begin (or end) a JMT hike if you cannot get a permit for Whitney Portal. See elevation profile below and maps on the previous four pages.

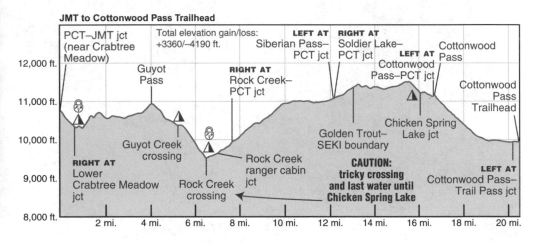

JMT to Cottonwood Pass Trailhead

Ranger Stations and Emergency Contacts

RANGER CABIN LOCATIONS IN SEQUOIA AND KINGS CANYON NATIONAL PARKS

Ranger Cabin (Distance from HI/WP)	GPS Coordinates Where You Leave JMT	GPS Coordinates of Ranger Cabin
McClure Meadow (Section 7; 119.9/102.3)	37.188062°N, 118.743837°W	37.188004°N, 118.742886°W
How to get there: Head 300 feet northeast of the trail, along the stretch of McClure Meadow with many campsites; easily missed when headed south.		
Le Conte Canyon (Section 8; 137.8/84.4)	37.094135°N, 118.594327°W	37.093835°N, 118.595000°W
How to get there: Head 200 feet west on the spur trail at the Dusy Basin/Bishop Pass junction.		
Bench Lake, * ** (Section 9; 159.0/63.2)	36.961496°N, 118.438871°W	36.961528°N, 118.437587°W
How to get there: From between the Taboose Pass and Bench Lake junctions, head 350 feet due east to the canvas-sided ranger cabin.		
Rae Lakes (Section 10; 175.6/46.6)	36.811291°N, 118.400814°W	36.810931°N, 118.400047°W
How to get there: Located toward the northern end of the middle of the three Rae Lakes. Head 250 feet southeast along the spur trail.		
Charlotte Lake (Section 11; 180.8/41.4)	36.770634°N, 118.416255°W	36.777324°N, 118.426082°W
How to get there: From Sandy Junction on the JMT, head 0.9 mile northwest on the trail to Charlotte Lake. The ranger cabin is just east of the trail, toward the northern end of the lake.		
Tyndall Creek* (Section 12; 195.6/26.6)	36.639849°N, 118.388239°W	36.632574°N, 118.391959°W
How to get there: Head 0.6 mile southwest on the trail descending Tyndall Creek. The cabin is just west of the trail.		
Crabtree (Section 12; 204.1/18.1)	36.564793°N, 118.350404°W	36.564732°N, 118.347305°W
How to get there: Head south across Crabtree Creek to the Crabtree camping area. Then walk 0.1 mile east along a spur trail to the cabin.		
Rock Creek (along PCT south of JMT)	36.495876°N, 118.329695°W	36.495408°N, 118.326455°W
How to get there: Head 0.2 mile east along a spur trail to the cabin.		

* These stations are sometimes unmanned due to budgetary limitations.
** The Bench Lake station is a canvas tent that is assembled when the station is staffed. The platform is not visible from the JMT when the cabin is down.

EMERGENCY CONTACTS

JURISDICTION	TRAIL SECTION (Mileage from Happy Isles)	PHONE NUMBERS
Yosemite NP	Yosemite Valley to Donohue Pass (0–36.1 miles)	209-379-1992
Inyo County Sheriff	Donohue Pass to Island Pass (36.1–41.3 miles)	760-878-0383
Madera County Sheriff	Island Pass to Madera–Fresno County Line (near Deer Creek) (41.3–64.2 miles)	559-675-7770
Devils Postpile NM	Devils Postpile NM (57.0–58.9 miles)	760-934-2289
Fresno County Sheriff	Madera–Fresno County Line to Piute Bridge (64.2–112.1 miles)	559-488-3111 (only for outside Kings Canyon NP)
Sequoia and Kings Canyon NP	Piute Bridge to Mount Whitney (112.1–213.7 miles)	559-565-3195 or 559-565-3341
Inyo County Sheriff	Trail Crest to Whitney Portal (213.7–222.2 miles)	760-878-0383

About the Author

ELIZABETH WENK has hiked and climbed in the Sierra Nevada since childhood and continues the tradition with her husband, Douglas Bock, and daughters, Eleanor and Sophia. As she obtained a PhD in Sierran alpine plant ecology from the University of California, Berkeley, her love of the mountain range morphed into a profession.

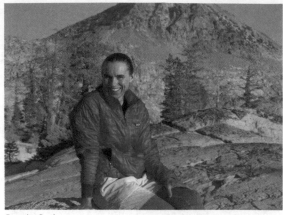

Douglas Bock

Writing guidebooks has become her way to share her love and knowledge of the Sierra Nevada with others. Lizzy continues to obsessively explore every bit of the Sierra, spending summers hiking on- and off-trail throughout the range, but she currently lives in Sydney, Australia, during the off-season. Other Wilderness Press titles she has authored or coauthored include *Yosemite National Park: Your Complete Hiking Guide; Top Trails Yosemite; One Best Hike: Mount Whitney; One Best Hike: Grand Canyon; Backpacking California; Sierra North; Sierra South; 50 Best Short Hikes: Yosemite;* and *Wildflowers of the High Sierra and John Muir Trail,* a perfect companion book for all naturalists.

Lizzy is also a board member of the John Muir Trail Wilderness Conservancy, a foundation dedicated to the preservation of the JMT corridor and surrounding High Sierra lands.